RADIONICS AND RADIESTHESIA

A Guide to Working with Energy Patterns

JANE E. HARTMAN

Foreword by

LUTIE LARSON
GLADYS T. MCGAREY

New Age Books

ISBN: 81-7822-166-7

First Indian Edition: Delhi, 2004

(Previously published 1999 by Aquarian Systems, Publishers, USA)

(Originally published as *Shamanism for the New Age: A Guide to Radionics & Radiesthesia* 1987)

Disclaimer:

Neither the author nor the publisher accepts any responsibility whatsoever for effects that may result from following the remedial and other techniques described herein. Nor do they make any claims, medical or otherwise, concerning the efficacy of this material.

Published by

NEW AGE BOOKS

A-44 Naraina Phase-I

New Delhi-110 028 (INDIA)

Email: nab@vsnl.in

Website: www.newagebooksindia.com

Printed in India

at Shri Jainendra Press

A-45 Naraina Phase-I, New Delhi-110 028

To my students—

May you be always

in the Light

Contents

List of Figures

Foreword to the New Edition

Radionics and radiesthesia have for a long time been considered metaphysical sciences. I like to define *metaphysical* as "beyond physical." Metaphysics, although referring to phenomena we all know about, describes the invisible. When something is invisible, we can't see it, yet we sometimes feel it is actually there. Air, for example, is invisible, but when there is a breeze, we can feel it. Although we don't know what air looks like or understand exactly what it is, we know it is important to us.

The sciences of radionics and radiesthesia allow us to begin to understand a variety of invisible phenomena. What is it, for instance, that causes a seed to germinate, sprout, and grow? What causes a plant to blossom and set fruit that carries within it the seed of the next generation? These processes, like the movement of air, are invisible to us; we see only their results. Every once in a while the wonder of such phenomena catches our attention, although most of the time we take the phenomena themselves for granted.

By the early 1900s, a few scientists had focused their attention on this invisible aspect of living forms—the "something" that comes first and the "something" that maintains the physical form. They were especially fascinated by the idea that an ordered set of instructions has the responsibility of maintaining the physical forms we think of as us.

Through careful observation, these scientists discovered that "parts" of a physical form would eventually break down, losing their integrity, their strength, and ultimately their definition. Why the breakdown into degeneration and disease? Because subtle energy fields had become confused and the "instructions" had failed to establish a link with the physical. What's more, the scientists noted that the *dis-ease conditions* seemed to have specific patterns, or waveforms, that, if allowed to persist, interrupted and caused distortions in *healthy subtle fields.*

Radionic researchers found that once they were able to link a disease pattern with a particular waveform setting on a resonant instrument, they could use this setting to reestablish healthy patterns in people, animals, plants, soil, or environments. This model for healthy maintenance of the physical life-form catapulted the newly developed radionic technique into practical use in health care and agriculture. The science of radionics thus became a way to "feel the breeze" and ultimately "see" the invisible.

The science of radiesthesia came into being soon after it was recognized that the human form is an ideal "antenna" and the human mind is capable of recognizing a variety of complex waveforms. The radiesthesic method of linking with subtle patterns entails an operator and a dowsing device—usually a pendulum. The operator uses his mind to scan for specific patterns in the subtle fields of an organized life-form. Upon recognizing one of these patterns, he proceeds to measure it, ask questions about it, and focus on the causes behind the precipitating condition. As for the dowsing device, it is simply a bob, or weight of any sort, suspended on a string or chain held between the fingers. Its movement indicates the presence or absence of a field resonant with the waveform produced by the operator's thought.

The various settings, or "rates," on a radionic instrument are each linked with a subtle field. When activated, they send out waveform patterns that "tune" their respective fields. Such an instrument thereby acts as an interface, allowing the operator to both observe and "harmonize" the subtle fields, releasing any distorting patterns.

The study of subtle energy actually began centuries ago. German physician Franz Mesmer (1734–1815), German poet and science writer Johann Wolfgang von Goethe (1749–1832), and British physicist Ernest Rutherford (1871–1937), among other researchers, all noticed the existence of something beyond the physical form—something attached to, or otherwise associated with, the physically manifested organism. Interestingly, the more attention investigators gave to these subtle forces, the more perceptible the forces became, and the more appreciated as well.

Our own awareness of the subtle aspects of our being triggers an experience of the multidimensional layers of life. In *The Findhorn Garden,* a book by the Findhorn community in northern Scotland, we find this counsel from the apple tree deva: "As from the seed a tree grows, so from the seed idea a pattern [waveform] issues forth . . . . Growing in strength and size, the pattern becomes brighter until eventually it scintillates and sounds. . . . This is the word made flesh, held in balance by great layers of life."

If we truly understood how moment to moment our physical world comes into be-ing, wonder would lift us high and we would marvel at the miracle of life. Working with radionics and radiesthesia brings us to this threshold by opening our consciousness. Reality as we know it expands, and our world seems much more wondrous than we could have imagined while perceiving only the physical.

LUTIE LARSEN
Longtime radionic researcher, teacher, former
vice president of the United States Psychotronics
Association, and publisher of the bimonthly
Radionic Homestead Report

Foreword to the Original Edition

My first conscious awareness of energy patterns in relationship to medicine takes me back to my childhood in India. One bright, sunny morning when I was ten years old, I was called away from the breakfast table because a snake charmer had presented himself in front of my family's bungalow in Northern India. He had apparently been out the night before, had found a new cobra, was unable to remove its fangs, and now wished to show it to my father. My parents, both physicians, were very interested in Indian customs, so we went to observe the performance.

The moment we arrived, the snake charmer told the crowd to stand back. Then he picked up a flat basket. As he lifted the basket's lid, a cobra slithered out so fast that before the man was able to reach for his flute, handmade from a gourd and bamboo pipes, the cobra had slid nearly fifteen feet away from him.

When the snake charmer began to play his flute, the creature stopped, raised its body in the air, opened its hood, and with a gentle swaying motion, slid back to the snake charmer, as if attached to him by an invisible string. As the man continued to play, the snake, hypnotized by the music, kept inching forward. The moment the music stopped, however, the cobra struck at him. The man, catching the snake under the chin, flipped it back, picked up his flute, and started playing again. This happened several more times until the cobra, outpacing the snake charmer, bit him on the index finger.

Instantly, the fun and games ended. The snake charmer quickly threw a blanket over the snake and, wrapping the creature up, returned it to the basket. He then tied a root around his upper arm, forming a tourniquet, reached into a container filled largely with herbs, and took out a small black stone. By then, his entire arm was shaking visibly and he had broken out in a sweat, all the while coughing uncontrollably. No sooner did he place the black stone on his injured finger than it seemed to "attach itself" to his wound. After ten or fifteen minutes, the stone dropped to the ground, at which point the man's hacking and sweating subsided. He proceeded to pick up the stone, tap it on the gourd, and watch while several drops of yellow fluid oozed out of his finger, staining the gourd. Finally, he announced that he was going to be all right.

For decades later this phenomenon raised tantalizing questions in my mind: What had caused the cobra to stop and work its way back to the snake charmer? Although the flute music was certainly not melodious to my ears, could it have sent out a vibration or energy pattern that somehow mesmerized the snake? And what had kept the small black stone fastened to the snake charmer's finger until it had drawn the venom from his system, assisting his recovery from an otherwise potentially fatal bite?

Unanswered questions like these have posed mysteries for many of us. In the pages that follow, Dr. Hartman presents concepts and ways of developing the senses that help us understand such puzzling energy patterns. Although all the answers are certainly not yet in, this volume brings together many of those that are. Best of all, it spells out how to use the material in working with our own energy patterns, those of others, and those present in the environment around us.

I highly recommend this book as a source of information for the seeker.

GLADYS T. MCGAREY, MD, MDH

Introduction

When this book was originally written more than eleven years ago, many twentieth-century seers believed that the time was fast approaching when Mother Earth would cleanse herself in earnest, drastically changing life as we know it. Some of the more dire predictions had us going the way of the woolly mammoth. Today, closer as we are to the predicted changes, it appears that even if only a few of them come to pass we may be forced to rely on our inner resources to survive. Hence, I have felt compelled to update and revise this guide to working with energy patterns.

Preparation for dramatic earth and infrastructure changes has been the subject of an avalanche of books, videos, and articles. Each one suggests that surviving without water treatment plants, electrical systems, or even the uncountable luxuries we have become accustomed to will not be easy. Accomplishing such a feat, we are told, will require us to exercise our intuitive powers. Expertise is often born of necessity, and if the seers are on target, the skilled use of intuition may well be our saving grace.

A large body of evidence indicates that human reliance on intuitive faculties is nothing new. For centuries American Indian medicine people have known how to be in tune with the earth and how to use the powers inherent in this attunement. Indeed, indigenous people everywhere once recognized themselves as part of a great unfolding consciousness that served as a source of inner knowing.

Utilizing similar techniques, our tribal ancestors around the world enlisted energies from other dimensions to help with survival, and for healing purposes as well. Many of these people regarded supernatural forces as real and viable parts of everyday life. Poised between the visible and invisible worlds, they called on animal spirits and other totem beings to act as guardians, protectors, or guides. Often, these helpers fostered our forebears' survival by manipulating universal energies and by assisting in the selection of colors, stones, and other vibrationally healing agents. There is little doubt that to achieve and maintain these relationships, our progenitors entered into altered states ranging from deep trance to conscious knowing, all the while relying heavily on their intuitive powers.

The more recently established science of radionics is founded on similar principles, as you will see in the pages that follow. In this expanded edition you will find the most up-to-date remedies, color, gems, scents, and other means of transmitting specific vibrations to energize your healing faculties. In addition, you will learn the various patterns and circuitry needed for focusing your mind on analytical inquiries and therapeutic outcomes.

Serious radionic practitioners, like shamans old and new, alter their everyday consciousness and enter into an intuitive state to bring in needed information. As for its source, I shan't hazard a guess, although from considerable experience I can say that much of this information does not come from the conscious mind or diligent studies. I, for one, experience directing energies that are at times quite strong, as well as the presence of angelic guides. Indeed, many radionic practitioners have had visionary or inspired moments, and routinely rely on what Australian Aborigines term "the strong eye"; we "imagine" and visualize as a matter of course. Unlike our predecessors, however, we base our practice on a methodology with a proven track record.

Through the techniques described in this book, you will learn to utilize your finely tuned nervous network—one of the best engineered systems in the world—as both a diagnostic and a treatment tool. You will also learn to tap into the same innate abilities exhibited by early healers and to direct the powers of your mind for purposes of promoting harmony and well-being.

These techniques are only a beginning, however. The true student of this work will be entranced, as I have been, by the limitless nature of its applications. So follow your creativity as far as it will lead you, then step beyond it, into the world of unlimited energies. At that point your perceptions will be forever enhanced. As Oliver Wendell Holmes once said, "A mind stretched by a new idea can never go back to its original dimensions."

Acknowledgments

My sincere thanks to the following for permission to quote from publications or to reproduce materials: Perry Coles, president of the Lucis Trust (Alice A. Bailey books, especially *Esoteric Psychology I & II, Esoteric Healing, A Treatise on Cosmic Fire,* and *A Treatise on White Magic*); Mrs. Jean Westlake Cormack, daughter of Dr. Aubrey T. Westlake (the Static Diamond pattern); Dr. Christopher Hills and the University of the Trees Press (the Magnetron pattern); Dr. Hazel R. Parcells (Parcells's Evaluation Sheet); the Radionic Association of Great Britain, Vicki Roberts, editor of *Radionic Quarterly,* and John Walker, chairman (definition of radionics); Aart Jurriaanse of South Africa for writing *Bridges;* Hedda Lark at DeVorss & Co. (*Through the Curtain* by V. P. Neal and S. Karagulla); John Pasmantier at Grove Press (*The Science of Homeopathy* by George Vithoulkas); The Theosophical Publishing House of Madras, India, and Wheaton, Illinois (*The 7 Human Temperaments* by Geoffrey Hodson); C. W. Daniel Co., Ltd. (*Chakras, Rays and Radionics* by David V. Tansley, *An Introduction to Medical Radiesthesia and Radionics* by V. D. Wethered, and *Aluminum Utensils and Disease* by H. Tomlinson, MD); Harper & Row (*The Way of the Shaman* by Michael Harner and *Seven Arrows* by Hyemeyohsts Storm); Aquarian Press, Thorson's Publishing Group Ltd. (*The Seven Rays* by Dr. Douglas Baker); Routledge & Kegan Paul (*The Raiment of Light* by David V. Tansley); and Skip Gordon at Rudolf Steiner Press.

Also, my gratitude and love to the following for their assistance, encouragement, and permission: Mrs. Margaret Belsham at Magneto Geometric Applications in England for her gracious assistance over the years (analysis form and Malcolm Rae quote); Dr. John Hyslop, president of the Sathya Sai Baba Council of America (quotations from discourses and sayings of Sri Sathya Sai Baba); Dr. Jean G. Brown for invaluable technical assistance and support; Roslyn Eisenberg for editorial help and advice; Anita Hight-Perry for art and graphics; Chad Perry for his professional editing skills; Allachaquora for her gem therapy expertise; and Nancy Long, Virginia Lampson, Elizabeth Nachman, Richard Katz, Ann McIntyre, and the many others who have encouraged me to write it all down.

A very special thank you to Dr. Gladys T. McGarey and to Brooke Medicine Eagle for taking time out of their busy lives to struggle through the intial galleys and make valuable contributions to the first edition of this book.

In conclusion I would like to thank the teachers, colleagues, and friends who contributed to the vast amount of material added to this new edition: Poonam and Vinvd Nagpal from India's Sai Sanjeevini Foundation & Trustees; Michael Blate, executive director of the G-Jo Institute, for his help and guidance; Lutie Larsen, for her invaluable update on radionically supported agriculture; Shelley Donnelly, for her fascinating work in Pranamonics; Oceana Lowry, for her innovative color work; Erla Mae Larson and Jean Kinne, for invaluable assistance; and the exciting editorial and production team headed by incredible Ellen Kleiner. I love you all!

Credits

The following contributions were written specifically for this edition:

Chapter 1

The Nature of Energy Systems

Microcosms of the Universe

Field is the only reality.
—Albert Einstein

Everything that exists is a form of energy—you, the neighbor's dog, a tree, a rock, a table, even the book you are reading. In other words the molecular structure of all life, from animate to inanimate, is in constant motion. Matter, which is energy confined to physical form, represents the densest type of energy. It has been said by students of ageless wisdom that matter is spirit at its lowest level of cyclical activity, whereas spirit is matter at its highest.

Accepting the notion that everything is energy moves us beyond the first barrier to manipulating energy systems. To cross the next obstacle, we must come to see that what essentially distinguishes us from a table, or a rock in the garden, is our energy's rate of vibration. If we were as accomplished as some yogis and able to increase the frequency of our energy, we would have no trouble passing our hands through a table.

Legitimate psychic healers from the Philippines—a multitude of charlatans also abound—can, through certain ritual procedures including prayer and biblical readings, elevate their vibrational rates enough to pass their hands through human flesh. This practice is mind-boggling to many Westerners, but only because we have not yet learned to view matter as energy.

Seeing Matter As Energy

In contemplating the elements of our world—earth, air, fire, and water—we tend to bypass all notions of energy. Consider an ice cube, for example. Frozen, it is solid; melted, it turns to liquid; boiled, it converts to gas. Viewing our world in terms of solids, liquids, and gases, we immediately separate matter into its manifest forms. Yet in the case of the melting ice cube, the same chemical components of hydrogen and oxygen have simply expressed themselves in different vibrational rates. By thinking in terms of energy, we would grasp this essential oneness underlying the forms we observe.

One way to begin is to perceive the human body as a universe. Early philosophers in fact called the body a microcosm of the macrocosm. Second-century German visionary St. Hildegard of Bingen, among numerous others, gave voice to this perception when she pleaded, "Oh, man, look at man! For man has in himself heavens and earth."

Even at the cellular level, we represent a universe. And within this orderly cosmos, everything from an orbiting comet to the formation of two new nuclei vibrates rhythmically. The atoms themselves, with their circling electrons, each resemble a solar system of planets revolving about a nucleus.

Another way to envision the body is as a musical chord in which each organ produces a distinctive note. Despite their differing frequencies, they vibrate in harmony.

We are usually unaware that the human body is vibrating. Upon closer examination, however, we can see that every material part of us is in a state of oscillation. Each cell, for instance, is like a small battery; within its atoms, positively and negatively charged electric particles interact, producing the energy needed to propel the cell on its life course. The individual atoms, for their part, all vibrate at their own rates and combine to form molecules of varying frequencies. In the end, the rate at which a cell vibrates is the sum of the frequencies of its components.

The body's cells take on unique characteristics as they converge into organs such as the stomach and heart, each of which has its own vibrational rate. This rate is subject to change as the organ's cellular makeup changes—that is, as the constituent cells undergo the natural process of birth, growth, death, and dissolution.

To function effectively, *all parts of the human body must be in harmony.* If vibrations are disturbed in any portion of the body, the disturbance will affect the entire organism, resulting in dis-order, or dis-ease. A state of disorder can also arise in response to an external influence, such as a person who increases our level of discomfort. The scientific explanation for this phenomenon is "incompatibility of frequencies." Such instances of dis-ease are attributed to the coming together of two energy systems that are not in resonance—or in common parlance, meeting up with a person whose vibrations are "out of sync" with ours.

So it is that we, like everything else in the universe, are composed of one energy that manifests in a vast array of sometimes compatible and sometimes incompatible forms. Over the years this energy has been called everything from the odic force, or od, to orgone energy, the vital force, *prana,* the molecular ether, psychometric energy, God, It, or Manitou. Today, based on scientific documentation, we may conclude that the ultimate state of all matter is *primordial energy in motion.* In other words, what we perceive as solid is in truth a "hoax" perpetrated by our senses.

> *The energy with which the most elementary and subtle particles of matter are bound with each other is Divine. The individual separation of these energy particles is absolutely precise and cannot be altered by anyone. Any separation or merger would mean the nonexistence of Creation. The Divine Energy is God.*
>
> —Sri Sathya Sai Baba

The Characteristics of Energy Fields

Energy is expressed in so many ways that human consciousness, limited as it is, cannot grasp the full scope of it. We are familiar with energy expressed as form, but there is also what might be called finer energy, such as the formless "free" energy of electricity and thought that is often active in fields.

At the living system level, an invisible force has long appeared to guide all life functions. In the 1930s, former anatomy professor at Yale University School of Medicine Harold Saxon Burr identified this force as an energy field, providing well-documented evidence that energy fields do indeed exist around living things. Burr found that wherever there is life there are electrodynamic fields that can be measured and mapped. In over forty years of research into these life-fields (L-fields), his most transcendental discovery, however, was that their existence seems to *precede* the appearance of any trace of the physical forms to which they correspond. This finding suggests that energy fields do *not* emanate from preexisting physical structures, but rather serve as the organizing principle behind the appearance of these structures. L-fields, he noted, form the atoms into cells and condition them to perform certain functions. In short, L-fields are the blueprints of form.

Around the time that Burr was making his startling L-field discoveries, Russian researchers Senyon and Valentina Kirlian invented a technique for photographing these fields as they radiated outward from living things. Like Burr, the Kirlians found that illness could be predicted by changes appearing in a person's vital fields. Dr. Thelma Moss, a renowned expert in psi phenomena, began working extensively with Kirlian photography in the United States, where it was being used successfully in psychiatry as well. Other researchers showed that the L-fields of trees observed over a thirty-year period fluctuated in response to moon cycles and to the presence of sunspots, light, darkness, and storms. This work seemed to answer the question posed by scientists and metaphysical thinkers alike—namely, if we are all one energy, are we subject to a plethora of cosmic forces, as astrologers have been saying all along?

In the 1970s cardiologist-turned-mystic W. Brugh Joy, MD, found that Egyptian mummies appeared to have residual traces of an energy field. The fact that he could feel these vibrations with his sensitive hands indicated that energy fields may hover around the human form after death. How long such a field might remain has little bearing on our understanding since time and space are, like solid matter, inventions of the human mind.

Field itself is an ordered pattern that becomes manifest in a living system. It has been suggested that in addition to a life-field there is an organization field (O-field), which surrounds the universe, governing everything in it. This configuration is sometimes referred to as the O-field of the Creator, and at other times as a higher mind field.

In the 1930s psychiatrist Leonard J. Ravitz, MD, discovered that thought can affect the L-field, foreshadowing O. Carl Simonton's use of thought focusing with cancer patients, which we now call positive imaging. In addition, Ravitz predicted that a thought-field (T-field) could probably attach to an energy field and, of all things, take a ride on it! Whereas it used to be said that "energy follows thought," we can now say, with confidence, that "thought *is* energy," and as such, thought is a viable force.

T-fields can attach not only to energy fields but also to *crystallized* forms of energy, or matter. A psychometrist holding an object, for example, can access everything that has happened to the object since it was produced—a practice resulting in many interesting tales about antiques and other historical items. When early Hawaiian priest-healers known as *kahunas* spoke of the *aka* threads connecting people to everything they have come in contact with since birth, perhaps they were referring to the means by which today's psychometrists are able to reveal their stories.

The observation that T-fields, or thought forms, can attach to other energies has enormous implications. For one, it suggests that a casual thought can set up a chain reaction with potentially disastrous consequences. For another, it implies that rather than formulating our thoughts, we *select* them from a "bank" in the ethers via a process governed by our condition at the time. Furthermore, the attachment property of T-fields intimates that the adage "Sticks and stones may break my bones, but words will never hurt me" is misleading, since words emanate from thought and thoughts can indeed hurt us.

As a result of the energy fields organizing the human body, all its functions are electrochemical. In addition, the cell's atomic substructure—that microscopic cosmos consisting of particles traveling faster than light—has magnetic moment, or the presence of a magnetic field. Hence, each cell can be viewed as possessing its own magnetic environment that combines with fields of other cells. Its magnetic properties result in part from the interaction of its electrochemical components.

Imagining a cell, we can visualize a constant transfer of electricity across its membranes, or borders. The electrical messages then carried along the nerves are determined by changes in the potassium (acid)/sodium-salt (alkaline) concentrations occurring on both sides of the borders; these changes, in turn, alter the cell's magnetic environment. A balance in the acid-alkaline levels of cells is therefore basic to the harmonious functioning of the human body. Similarly, a lack of harmony will show up as an imbalance in these levels. To avoid trouble in either direction, the acid-alkaline balance must be maintained. When it is not, the therapeutic use of magnetism, now practiced increasingly in Europe, can help reestablish the needed ratios.

Ultimately, humans can be impacted at the cellular level in two ways: through chemical action (via the ingestion of substances such as drugs) and through disruption of the electromagnetic frequency (by way of interaction with another field). In the latter instance, the body as an energy field will react to anything that emits radiation. In other words, the body's harmony can be disrupted by *all life forms.* The heartening news is that the state of harmony can be reestablished through magnetic realignment.

Here's how this works. Interestingly, more than 80 percent of the human body is composed of water (H_20). Although the oxygen (O) nucleus of water has no magnetic moment and does not on its own respond to external magnetic fields, the single proton of the hydrogen (H) nucleus is highly susceptible to such influences. As a result, water is easily polarized by an external magnetic field. And sure enough, the hydrogen protons in the body's water do realign themselves in response to an applied magnetic field.

Points to Remember

In this opening chapter we have addressed many aspects of energy systems. The major insights to carry into the material to come are as follows:

- All that is, is energy, and every form of energy vibrates at a rate determined by its components.
- All matter known to have oscillating charges radiates magnetic waves. Since everything contains electrons in motion, everything radiates magnetic waves. With this in mind, you might picture the entire universe as a vast array of pulsating electromagnetic fields, with everything from an atom to the stars participating in the cosmic dance. The pulsations produce two opposing forces, such as the North and South Poles of the earth, through the dynamics of attraction and repulsion, also known as ebb and flow, or yin and yang. The resulting polarity extends throughout our universe and beyond.
- Energy and matter are two aspects of the same reality. From an esoteric perspective, begin to think of reality as consciousness, and energy (including thought forms) and matter as its aspects.

> *The myriad songs of the universe are the Songs of Life. All energies dancing through the universe, and through interplay and movement, create a vast symphonic composition—mathematical in its precision, as music is mathematical, creative in its effect.*
>
> —Viola Petitt Neal and Shafica Karagulla

Chapter 2

Our Invisible Bodies

Cues to Our Physical Selves

> *Man is the manifestation in physical matter of the spiritual Monad, a single spark of the One Spirit.*
>
> —Aart Jurriaanse

As we continue to explore the invisible aspects of human health and disease, we are led to the importance of the subtle bodies. The subtle nature of humankind has been addressed by esoteric writings throughout the ages. Many of the answers we seek can be found there if only we have the patience to unravel this often confusing wellspring of material, and the desire to listen, adapt, and evolve as spirit dictates.

Perhaps the most lucid explanation of the subtle origins of humans appears in a book entitled *Bridges* by Aart Jurriaanse, an authority on Alice A. Bailey's thirty years of channeling Tibetan master DK, beginnning in 1919. These channelings present what many people regard as a core explanation of the subtle forces guiding human constitution and evolution. *Bridges* provides a highly informative shortcut to understanding the sometimes complicated Bailey volumes, although serious students will want to study the work of both authors.

In keeping with the scope of his efforts, Jurriaanse has dedicated *Bridges* to "Humanity without reservation," adding, "Man's version of the Truth should not be offered with restrictions." In a chapter entitled "The Planes of Existence" he has described the physical plane as encompassing the four lower kingdoms of mineral, vegetable, animal, and human—that is, all dense matter. Here we learn that although humans are conditioned to focus on the substantial aspects of this plane, beyond its solid, liquid, and gaseous states can be found a more subtle realm known as the *etheric body,* which is not normally perceptible to humans. And beyond the etheric body are other insubstantial worlds, all forming a bridge to the spiritual plane.

Invisible Bodies on the Physical Plane

In addition to the etheric body, which is addressed in detail in the second half of this chapter, there is the *astral body,* or emotional body, often called the desire body. We tend to engage our energies in this sphere of glamour, distraction, illusion—in short, in the alluring traps of the material world. Most human dis-ease takes root here, as well. The vibration of the astral body reflects the individual's degree of attractiveness and therefore carries psychic implications. Many sensitives, for example, contact the astral plane to access information. I once asked a knowledgeable man about the risks involved in accepting information from anything other than the finer spiritual planes, to which he replied, "Dying doesn't give you the smarts!"

In earlier times the astral body kept human beings multiplying and evolving. Today, as energies are becoming more refined, its function is changing.

At the highest level of the physical plane is the *mental body.* (*Note:* "higher" and "lower" in this context refer to humans' evolution toward perfection.) The mental body is made of mind stuff—in Sanskrit, *chitta*—and is the most subtle of the physical energies. The mental vibration, by means of the will, seeks to coordinate the function of the physical body and thereby impacts on physical well-being. Although it strives to link up the lower self with higher consciousness, it can also repulse these finer energies and cause separation. Together, the mental, astral, and physical bodies make up the personality.

The personality level of consciousness is the only one we are normally aware of. As we evolve and open to higher consciousness levels, however, we become able to enhance our awareness of the more subtle "transpersonal" spiritual planes. These consist of, in ascending order, *intuition,* or the soul, also known as the higher self, the ego, and the Christ within; *spirit,* or innermost essence of the individual; *the monad,* which reflects universal order; and *divinity* itself.

So it is that the human constitution spans the planes, from physical to spiritual, as depicted below.

Transpersonal Aspects—Spiritual Plane
Divine body of deity
Monadic body
Spiritual or atmic body
Intuitional or Buddhic (soul) body

Personality—Physical Plane
Mental body
Astral/Emotional body
Etheric/Physical body

Functions of the Etheric Body

Our origin as dense physical beings is in a complex mass of forces and fields in the first cosmic ether (see figure 2–1). As it is said in the Vedas, sacred writings of ancient India: "What is the origin of this world? Ether . . . for all these beings take their rise from the ether only, and return into the ether. Ether is greater than these; ether is their rest."

Hence, surrounding and interpenetrating the physical body is the etheric body, also called the vital body. It is known, too, as the etheric double, because it mirrors and appears to conform to the physical body. A web of its energy holds together the subtle forms of the personality.

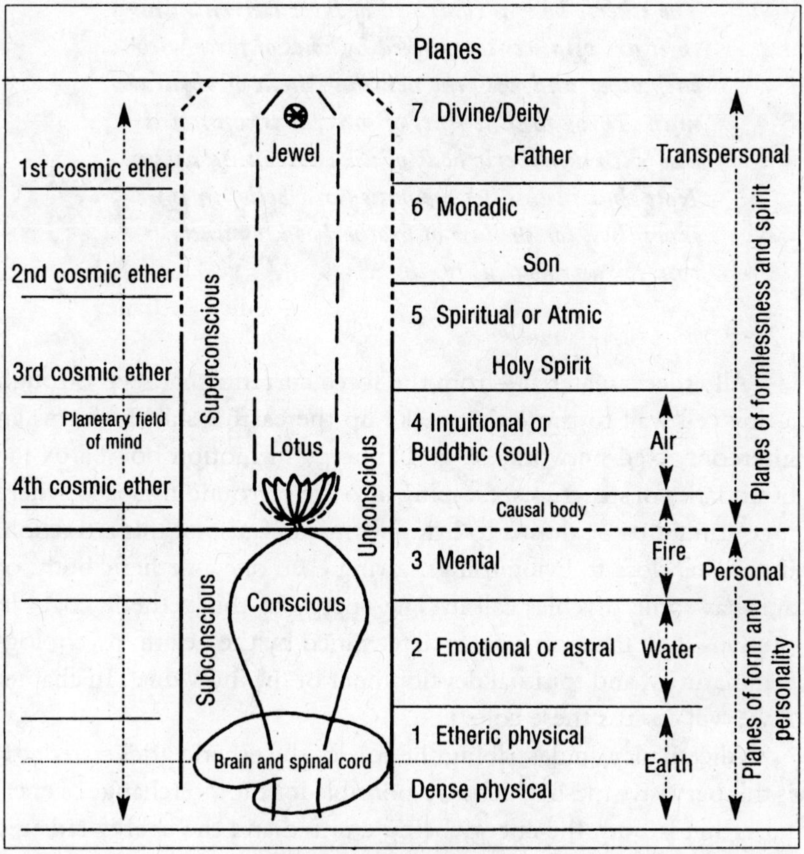

Adapted from a diagram presented in a lecture by Dr. Elmer Green (1972)

Figure 2–1 Interpretation of the Human Constitution

> *The etheric body is composed of force currents and in it are vital centers linked by lines of force with each other and with the nervous system of physical man. Through these lines of force, it is connected also with the etheric body of the environing system. Note that in this lies the basis for a belief in immortality, for the law of brotherhood, or unity, and for astrological truth.*
>
> —Alice A. Bailey

All etheric material—from the force currents that seep through a tiny cell wall to those that make up the earth's shield—forms an interconnected network, or grid. Energy in motion bombards the boundaries of structures, escaping into the surrounding space, where it continues to be drawn to living forms. Because of this attraction, it remains close to living things, giving each one an etheric body, or aura, as some psychics call it. The energy of this "etheric coat" in humans then takes on a color determined by the health, psychological maturity, and spiritual development of the individual. In chapter 8 we will discuss these colors.

Alice Bailey, in describing the role of the etheric grid, stated: "It is this pervasive mesh which is responsible for the interchange of energies, that is both the energy being emitted and the energy radiated and the energies being absorbed from external energy sources, which will exert their influence on the form. The etheric web or network underlies the nervous system in living things." Indeed, the etheric body is the foundation and framework on which the material body is constructed.

What gives rise to the physical nervous system is an etheric one composed of subtle channels known as *nadis,* Sanskrit for motion. Arthur Avalon (Sir John Woodroffe), foremost student of Tantric texts, has compared the uncountable numbers of nadis associated with a human being to a complicated "chart of ocean currents." These subtle channels, which serve as conduits for the flow of *prana*—Sanskrit for life force—pass tentaclelike through the etheric spine and its power centers, called chakras, which we will explore in the next chapter.

The etheric body, with its nadis of flowing *prana*, constitutes the most vital part of the physical body's response mechanism. Essentially, it performs three functions: energy reception, energy assimilation, and energy transmission. This activity takes place not only in the etheric body's contact with the world of matter and human senses but also in its relationship with the higher astral and mental bodies. In this respect the etheric body is also a channel for developing expanded states of consciousness, which in times to come may well be its most important function.

In addition, the etheric body serves as a mirror—reflecting the state of the physical body on the one hand and of the mental and astral bodies on the other. A lack of harmony anywhere in the world of form will reflect in the etheric realm. In fact, disorder at the higher levels will register in the etheric body *before manifesting as a physical dysfunction*.

Etheric material exists in and around every form in our solar system and beyond. As a result, this giant network of interconnecting and interpenetrating force fields unites us with all of existence. The ultimate significance of this all-encompassing etheric web, a far leap from the work of Burr and other scientists, can be too staggering to contemplate. All we need to understand at this point is that any action occurring along the etheric network—from within it or outside it—will leave an imprint and trigger a reaction.

In other words, the universal law of cause and effect, or action and reaction, governs the channels of the etheric network. This means that whatever acts on one part of the etheric web will provoke a response in another part—which may then spark repercussions on the spiritual, mental, astral, or physical levels, if not all of them.

So it is that the etheric body operates as a register, or data bank, to which healers must direct their attention. Indeed, in the practice of radionics, this vital vehicle is a sphere of primary focus. In Alice Bailey's words: "All disease, barring mechanical injury and accident, originates in the subtle bodies. Therefore, a thorough understanding of their function and place in the human constitution is necessary for all practitioners. Think of the etheric body as a shimmering body of light, a reflection of the conditions of all the other subtle bodies, and the network that connects to the physical body. It is here that we find the key."

Chapter 3

Chakras and the Endocrine Glands

From Subtle Energy to Physical Structure

The lotus is a flower that has its roots in the mud (the material world); its stem grows up through the water (the astral or emotional world); and the bloom rising above the water into the air (the realm of mind) provides an excellent metaphor for the chakras.

—David V. Tansley

A line from the Upanishads—discourses on the deep wisdom of ancient India—states, "One cannot reach enlightenment without awakening and recognizing the chakras." Alice Bailey, in the early twentieth century, suggested that the etheric body and chakras through which it passes will be the next area of investigation in medical and scientific research. More recently Dr. Valerie Hunt, in her 1995 book *Infinite Mind,* explains that a former National Institutes of Health brain researcher who once applied a strictly neurochemical model to her work with neuropeptides and their receptors now "visualizes the brain and its functions as a vibratory energy field . . . [as] a receiver and amplifier of collective reality."

Some researchers, it appears, are already embarking on Alice Bailey's proposed mission. At the very least, they know that for healing to be effective the chakra systems must be understood. Hence, having examined the role of the etheric body in the previous chapter, we will now explore the interconnections between its energy centers—the chakras—and the energy-balancing function of their progeny, our endocrine glands.

Chakras, a Sanskrit word meaning wheels, are energy vortices. Many ancient writings compare them to lotus flowers bearing various numbers of petals and reflecting diverse states of unfolding. Seven major lotuslike configurations, together with at least twenty-one minor ones, are located along the etheric spine and about the head. Many more exist in other portions of the body, including several that correspond with important acupuncture points. Based on years of research, W. Brugh Joy has included excellent diagrams of chakra locations in his book *Joy's Way.*

The difference between the major and minor chakras is related to the number of crisscrossing lines of force passing through them. The more intersecting lines these centers have, the more powerful they are. Those with the most intersections are referred to as the seven major chakras.

It is the action of the chakras that transmits through the body the myriad energies surrounding us, including cosmic ones. In the words of radionic expert and esoteric scholar David V. Tansley: "Through these [chakras] the interplay of various energies build and sustain our endocrine glands and nervous system, and galvanize our organ systems into activity."

Basically, the chakras perform three functions: they vitalize the physical body, especially the endocrine glands and bloodstream; they enhance the consciousness of self; and they transmit spiritual energies, evoking states of spiritual beingness. Alice Bailey has described their action this way: "Chakras swirl astral, mental, and etheric material into activity, and their forces hold the physical form together."

These functions all occur simultaneously. In vitalizing the physical body, the chakras act as focal points for healing and balancing energies. Like powerful transducers of energies from within and without, they serve as radiating and distributing agents, each with a distinctive pattern of its own. In developing the consciousness of self, different chakras act in different ways. Those above the diaphragm, known as the higher chakras, open and become active as the individual progresses along a path of spiritual attunement; those below the diaphragm, reflecting a more primitive state of consciousness, tend to be already open and active. As for the transmission of spiritual energies, this task belongs solely to the higher power centers.

It is for good reason that these power centers are called "wheels," for they are often seen as whorls of concentric interblending energies, with colors that change as the condition of the system itself changes. Their vibrations vary, too; chakras above the diaphragm have higher frequencies than those below. Even the wheel-like rotation of the chakras can be influenced, especially by directed thought energy.

What determines the physical, emotional, and mental well-being of an individual is the *balanced functioning* of the chakras. In fact, most dis-eases can be traced to chakras that are out of balance. Because this is so, a practitioner investigating a physical disorder, for example, should as a matter of course check the chakra nearest the site of dysfunction to see if its energies are blocked, underactive, overactive, misdirected, or out of control. Defining the problem is step one in remediating it.

Properties of the Chakras

A closer examination of the major chakras, in all their uniqueness, can help us learn what they look like, how they operate, and what endocrine glands they govern. An awareness of this information is essential to any radionic analysis.

Figure 3–1, on page 17, shows the location and function of the chakras in a human being. You will note that this diagram illustrates not only the seven major vortices—the base, sacral, solar plexus, heart, throat, brow, and crown chakras—but also two additional ones, the spleen and alta major chakras. The *spleen chakra*, located near the physical spleen, has been added because it vitalizes the etheric body, and subsequently other power centers, by supplying them with *prana*, or life energy, including solar *prana* and planetary *prana*. Any unused *prana* is returned through this chakra's "gateway" to the etheric field

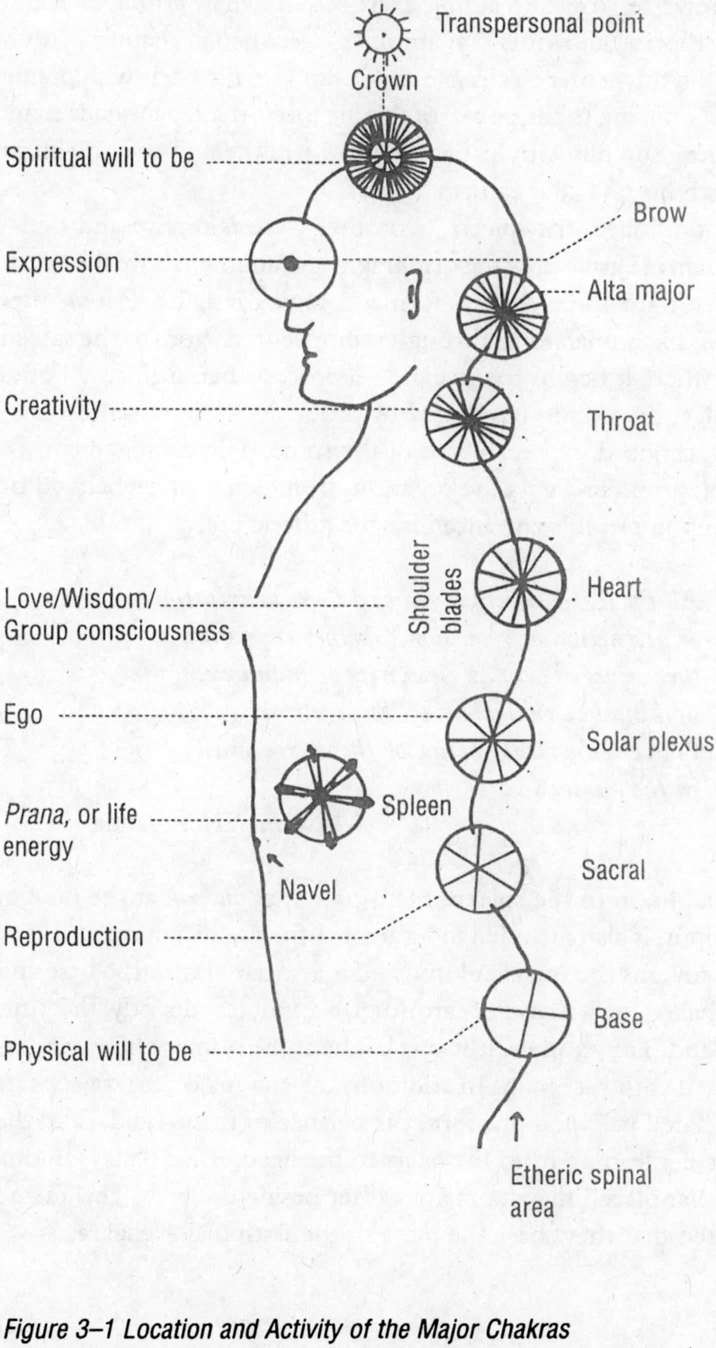

Figure 3–1 Location and Activity of the Major Chakras

of the universe. Yogic breathing exercises known as *pranayama* and the new therapy known as Pranamonics, described in chapter 7, both draw upon this center to cleanse and invigorate the body with pranic energy. Testifying to the power of this life force, the Upanishads state: "The rising sun fills with his rays all *pranas* in the universe and energizes with his rays all creatures."

In addition to the spleen, two other chakras receive and transmit *prana:* one just below the diaphragm and another above the heart. Together, these three vortices form a "pranic triangle." *Prana,* after accessing the human form through minor centers, goes to the spleen center, where it begins to circulate—a process that ordinarily bodes well unless the person is affected by problems in the seventh cervical and second dorsal vertebrae of the spine. This arrangement for handling *prana* prevents the organism from being overwhelmed by energy upon *prana*'s entrance into the etheric body.

> *All the forces, whether you call them gravitation or attraction or repulsion, whether expressing themselves as heat or electricity or magnetism, are nothing but variations of that unit energy. . . .* Prana *is the vital energy, or the source of all energy in the cosmos.*
>
> —Swami Vivekananda

In addition to the spleen, the *alta major chakra,* at the base of the occiput, is also included in figure 3–1 for significant reasons. For one, it governs the spinal column and is associated with the base and heart chakras, as well as the carotid gland and, less directly, the pituitary gland. For another, it is one of the three primary head centers associated with the brain. In addition, the alta major chakra appears to be related to blood pressure, the balance of tissue fluids, and the main artery leading from the heart to the head. Alice Bailey, among others, has placed the alta major center beside the brow chakra and suggested that they share the place of the sixth major chakra.

> *The brain is largely conditioned by three major glands which are found in close relation to the brain substance. These are the pituitary body, the pineal gland, and the carotid gland. These form a triangle, practically unrelated in primitive man, occasionally related in average man, and closely related in spiritual man. These glands are objective correspondences of the three energy centers by means of which the soul, or the indwelling spiritual man, controls his physical vehicle.*
>
> —Alice A. Bailey

Endocrine Glands—Next in the Chain of Command

The seven major centers externalize themselves as endocrine glands—ductless glands that empty their secretions directly into the bloodstream. Because of this activity, the endocrine glands are among the chief factors controlling well-being in the physical body. As externalizations of the chakras, they have a direct link with the etheric body. Hence, when these glands are in a state of balance, there is no disease in the physical organism and no obstruction to its more esoteric functions. In a sense, the endocrine glands form windows to most of the conditions encountered by practitioners.

Biochemical research has shown tremendous variability among the endocrine glands. Each one is distinct in its physiology and microscopic anatomy. These distinctions ultimately correspond to the conditions of the associated chakras as well as the individual endocrine patterns.

Relationships between the major chakras and their associated glands are outlined in figure 3–2. This chart, like the previous diagram, includes the spleen and alta major chakras. Here, too, you will see a number of lotus petals listed for each of the seven major chakras, a number that corresponds to the number and position of the nadis around it. In other words, the configuration of the nadis is what gives rise to each lotus-flower pattern.

Chakra (Sanskrit name)	Description	Location
1. Base, or root (*Muladhara*)	4-petaled lotus Red, gold	Base of spinal column between root of genitals and anus
2. Sacral (*Svadhisthana*)	6-petaled lotus Red, white	Midsacral region
3. Solar plexus (*Manipura*)	10-petaled lotus Black, dark blue, green, gold, red, gray	Below shoulder blades—in spine
4. Heart (*Anahata*)	12-petaled lotus Deep red, white, dark blue, yellow	Behind heart—in dorsal spine
5. Throat (*Visuddha*)	16-petaled lotus White, yellow, red to smoke	Base of throat
6. Brow (*Ajna*)	2-petaled lotus Intense white	Between eyebrows
7. Crown (*Sahasrara*)	1,000-petaled lotus Pattern leads to the Source White, red, yellow, black, green	Top of head
Spleen		Upper left side of abdomen
Alta major		Base of occipital bone

Figure 3–2 Chakra–Endocrine Gland Relationships

Function	Associated endocrine gland
Will to live on the physical plane; grounds to earth; directs life purpose; shelters Kundalini energy; animates substances of physical cells; governs kidneys, spine, nerves, dermis, chromofine tissue; energies transmute to crown for higher consciousness	Adrenals
Polarity chakra; guarantees species continuation; relates to ovaries, testes, uterus, all reproductive organs; governs sexual instincts; energies transmute to throat chakra for higher expression and balancing	Gonads
Seat of emotions; the ego; self-interest; clearinghouse for lower centers; dysfunction may be cause of cancer; digestive problems, skin problems, negativity, disharmony if overactive; governs liver, gall bladder, pancreas, digestive tract, sympathetic nervous system, abdominal viscera; energies transmute to heart chakra, center of group consciousness	Pancreas (Stomach)
Overstimulation may lead to heart problems; selfishness may lead to ulcers; aids response of adrenal cortex to stress; expresses love-wisdom, Christ- and Buddha-like qualities; center of group consciousness on highest and lowest levels; governs heart, blood, circulation, vagus nerve, immune system	Thymus
Higher intellect; will chakra; balance of power between reproduction and brain; the world of thought; governs vocal area, bronchial, lungs, digestive tract, throat, respiration	Thyroid/ Parathyroid
Overactivity may show other gland malfunction; center of integrated personality; third eye (higher mental clairvoyance); symbolizes world of life spirit; seat of mind; governs eyes, ears, nose, teeth, lower brain stem	Pituitary
Spiritual will to be; all-seeing eye of soul when awakened; possesses blueprints of all energy centers; seat of soul; world of divine spirit; balances will and love of God; contains replica of each chakra, hence the highly evolved will work through this chakra; governs brain, central nervous system	Pineal
Center of pranic reception and regulation; vitalizes physical body via bloodstream; manufactures white blood cells; stores iron	Spleen
Physical correspondence to *Antaskarana;* center of communication between the pineal and pituitary and vital energy of the spinal column (Kundalini); governs spinal column, carotid gland, tissue fluids, blood pressure	Pineal, pituitary, carotid (triangle of head centers' energies)

Many people experienced in esoteric studies and practices believe that the pineal and pituitary glands, both in the head triangle with the carotid, represent the individual's spirituality whereas the glands below the thyroid represent the lower self, or personality. In other words, they view the thyroid gland as a bridge between the two planes of human attainment. When referring to the glands in the head triangle, they associate the pineal with positive polarity and the pituitary with negative polarity, suggesting that their activity demonstrates a harmonious interplay of opposites.

Below are brief descriptions of the major glands, beginning with those most spiritually oriented. At the end of this section you will find information on glands associated with the spleen and alta major chakras.

Pineal

The pineal gland, associated with the crown chakra, is shaped somewhat like a pinecone. Attached to the roof of the third ventricle of the brain, it occupies a tiny "cave" behind and above the pituitary gland, where it acts as secretion director and general regulator of the other glands. Its own secretion—melatonin—seems to regulate the human bioclock. This gland also prevents early sexual maturation, tones muscles, influences skin pigmentation, and contributes to normal brain development.

Pituitary

This tiny, pea-shaped, two-lobed gland associated with the brow chakra is situated in the center of the head, at the base of the brain. Known as the "master gland," the pituitary helps regulate target glands. When they are working properly, it rests; if another gland is malfunctioning, however, the pituitary stimulates it with tropic hormone. Hence, when the pituitary is found to be overactive, other glands should be checked. The anterior and posterior lobes of the pituitary appear to independently stimulate the thyroid and adrenal glands, thereby affecting the energetics of the central nervous system, brain, and spinal cord. This gland also stimulates tissue growth, influences the sexual organs, and activates puberty.

Thyroid/Parathyroid

The thyroid gland, connected with the throat chakra, controls the overall growth of the body, oxidation processes, and mental development. It is extremely responsive to deep blue.

The parathyroid consists of four small glands located at the back lower edge of the thyroid gland, or sometimes embedded within it. They regulate the metabolism of phosphorus and calcium, affecting the neuromuscular system.

Thymus

The thymus gland, which is related to the heart center, appears to control normal bone growth and muscular metabolism during childhood. It strongly influences the adrenal cortex and its reaction to stress, as well as the pineal, thyroid, and prostate glands. Through its relationship to the heart center, the thymus gland is directly associated with the "thread of life" which, anchored in the heart, carries life energy throughout the body via the bloodstream. This gland also appears to influence the immune and autoimmune systems, and to activate the vagus nerve.

Pancreas

This gland, which is connected with the solar plexus chakra, performs a dual function: it regulates the production of insulin and secretes enzymes for digestion. Some authorities consider the stomach, too, to be an externalization of the solar plexus.

Gonads

The gonad glands, associated with the sacral chakra, help form the differentiated sex glands during embryonic development. Later serving as both the female sex glands (ovaries) and male sex glands (testes), they produce the cells needed for human reproduction—namely, the ova and spermatozoa. In the female, this gland internally secretes estrogen, which regulates and controls reproductive functions; in the male, it secretes the testosterone that stimulates metabolism and increases muscular strength.

Adrenals

The adrenal glands, linked with the base chakra, bring about the fight-or-flight response to danger. They also stimulate the growth of gray matter in the brain, the development of the sex cells, and the faculty for mental concentration and physical endurance. The adrenaline they secrete acts as a heart stimulant, reinforcing all-around well-being.

Spleen

Energetically, the spleen is the largest gland, although it is not recognized as such by modern medicine. The spleen manufactures white blood cells, stores iron, influences the nervous system, and aids in digestion. In radionics, the major function of the spleen is to supply the organism with *prana*, as described on page 18.

Pineal/Pituitary/Carotid

The three glands that correspond to the alta major center are all closely associated with the brain. In spiritually developed individuals, they transmit soul energy to the brain, which enables the soul to exert its influence over the personality.

Together, as crystallizations of their respective etheric bodies, these ductless glands control all the functions of the physical organism. Practitioners should therefore study the glands in depth. Knowledge of what they each do and how they do it is essential before working with the human energy field. And always, while interacting with the energetic chain of command between the subtle and physical structures of a human being, balance and coordination are the twin goals.

> *A man can be sick and ill, or well and strong, according to the state of the centers and their precipitation, the glands. It must ever be remembered that the centers are the major agency upon the physical plane through which the soul works, expresses life and quality, according to the point reached under the evolutionary process, and that the glandular system is simply an effect—inevitable and*

unavoidable—of the centers through which the soul is working. The glands, therefore, express fully the point in evolution of the man, and according to that point are responsible for defects or limitations, or for assets and achieved perfections. The man's conduct and behavior upon the physical plane is conditioned, controlled, and determined by the nature of his glands, and these are conditioned, controlled, and determined by the nature, quality, and the livingness of the centers; these in turn are conditioned, controlled, and determined by the soul, in increasing effectiveness as evolution proceeds. Prior to soul control, they are conditioned, qualified, and controlled by the astral body, and later by the mind. The goal of the evolutionary cycle is to bring about this control, this conditioning, and this determining process by the soul; human beings are today at every imaginable state of development within the process.

—Alice A. Bailey

Chapter 4

Dowsing for Health

The Pendulum As a Healing Tool

> *I believe profoundly that it is the privilege of radiesthesia [dowsing] to make its very special and, in some ways, unique contribution to the reintegration of material science and spiritual science, and to that restoration of wholeness of vision and outlook, of feeling and thinking which is the task of this age.*
>
> —Dr. Aubrey T. Westlake

Radiesthesia, the art and science of pendulum work, is a term coined by French priests in the early twentieth century. Dowsing itself, however, is over 5,000 years old. Feng shui masters in ancient China used this energy-monitoring technique to ensure that buildings were constructed in secure, earthquake-free, healthy areas. Pendulums and other dowsing instruments found in Egyptian tombs indicate that people of this ancient civilization relied on similar techniques. Early Celts and other earth-wise cultures also dowsed, primarily for water, minerals, and items encrusted in the soil.

The French priests who created the word *radiesthesia* advanced the practice from dowsing for water and minerals to dowsing for health, as they had become proficient in using the pendulum to locate diseases and prescribe remedies. The most well-known of these priests was Abbé Mermet whose classic work, *Principles and Practice of Radiesthesia*, was published in 1935. Mermet was considered the "king of dowsers" throughout Europe, including the Vatican, where his forty-year practice eventually established radiesthesia as a new science. In Europe radiesthesia remains a widely practiced discipline.

According to one of the many intriguing stories of Mermet's abilities, while in his study in Geneva, the Abbé accurately counted the number of railroad cars crossing a bridge over the River Seine in Paris, about 6,000 miles away! In addition to pinpointing this water source and monitoring the train traffic overhead, he provided correct geological information about the area. In his hand the pendulum was also used to solve crimes, treasure hunt, find missing people, analyze illnesses, and select proper remedies.

So it is that in the hand of a skilled operator whose mind has been cleared of all extraneous thoughts, a pendulum can detect the finest vibrations. Because such radiatory activity consists of measurable electromagnetic waves, the pendulum is regarded as an instrument of measurement. And because it allows our approximately thirty-seven miles of nervous system to tune into these subtle vibrations—some of which may as yet be unidentified by science—the pendulum can be viewed as an extension of our higher self, an extremely sensitive continuation of our human "antennae."

Proximity is of no account in detecting such subtle vibrations. Indeed space, as well as time, is merely a human construct. Like light waves—especially those at the ultraviolet end of the spectrum that travel at great speeds unimpeded by physical matter—radiesthetic rays are said to establish an almost instantaneous connection between a thought and the object of that thought. Actions at a distance, such as Abbé Mermet's detection of water 6,000 miles away, are said to occur as a result of the line of force projected by a thought, which can travel around the earth in one-seventh of a second.

The successful use of a pendulum therefore depends not on proximity, but rather on awareness. We, as operators, need only recognize that the universe is One, that everything and everyone in it has a unique vibrational rate we can tune into through our connection to the oneness.

> *The word* radiation *generally implies to the layman intangible, nonmaterial emanations given off by certain bodies. But to the physicist it means energy existing in electromagnetic waves. The word* influences *is used to denote nonmaterial forces as detected by the pendulum, and radiation indicates where the forces operate. Human sensitivity to these forces is registered by the pendulum. The human being seems to be a complex broadcasting station giving off radiations from every organ, tissue and structure. The pendulum deals with radiations thus detected and magnifies the effect.*
>
> —V. D. Wethered

Many people consider radiesthesia a type of halfway house between ordinary sense experience and extrasensory perception, placing it in a realm that physicist Christopher Hills has called "supersensonics." In fact, dowsing does rely on a supersense that makes direct contact with etheric formative forces and under certain circumstances with higher planes of existence. As a result of this interaction, a practitioner working with energies is able to detect oncoming dis-eases at subtle levels before they manifest in the gross physical vehicle.

> *There appear to be two sources of energy which produce the effects registered by the pendulum, or two schools of thought regarding it. One is that the energy is a part of the electromagnetic band and the human body is a mass of electrical forces. The other is that dowsing effects are metaphysical in nature, a product of the mind.*
>
> —H. Tomlinson, MD

Whichever school of thought you subscribe to, be sure to remember these two facts. First, all matter emits radiations; and second, every living being gives off electromagnetic waveforms that are indicative of its condition. In other words, the intensity and frequency of these vibrations reflect underlying psychological and physical factors. Consequently, any malfunction or disorder will be reflected in the electromagnetic waveforms and hence accessible to a radiesthethic practitioner.

Contemporary Uses of the Pendulum

The pendulum provides us with a measurement tool that is so sensitive it can pick up the finest vibrations from inert as well as active materials. In a sense it is akin to a radio, which translates oscillations into audible music; in the case of a pendulum, the ***human body*** is the translator.

Recent decades have given rise to a plethora of uses for pendulum work. Some of the more common ones are these:

- Searching for water, minerals, or geological formations. In 1949, for example, the well-known American dowser Harry Gross used a contour map of Bermuda while at his home in Maine to locate water on the islands. When the Bermuda authorities later drilled, they found water precisely where he said it would be. Prior to that time, their search for water had been unsuccessful.
- Surveying pipes, drains, and other water conduits to evaluate architectural sites for noxious radiation from underground waterways.
- Locating ley lines and power centers above and below the earth's surface.
- Archaeological site explorations.
- Medical and veterinary analyses and remedy selection.
- Horticultural and agricultural testing of soil, plant polarity, food vitality, and contamination from sprays or irradiation.
- Selecting homeopathic remedies and potencies.
- Finding lawbreakers, as well as missing people, animals, and property.
- Aptitude and personality assessment in personnel work, and biometric tests.
- Detecting harmful radiations in the air, water, and soil surrounding our living or work spaces.

In addition, dowsing is used to ascertain the causes of many conditions about which doctors and veterinarians have no fundamental knowledge. It has proved especially helpful to people who scurry from practitioner to practitioner, finding many remedies but no relief because the nature of their disorder has not been properly diagnosed. Harmful radiations or toxicity from subsoil, buried waste, or air pollutants are often implicated in such conditions, as are mercury, aluminum, or other metallic poisons. As H. Tomlinson, MD, states in his book *Aluminum Utensils and Disease: The Dangers Inherent in the Widespread Use of the Metal,* "Radiesthesia is the only science that fully explains the problem of aluminum poisoning, giving as it does the key to the whole matter, and enabling the physician to make an accurate diagnosis and prescribe suitable curative treatment."

Dowsing helps ascertain not only the cause of an ailment but also the site of the disturbance. A chart often used to dowse for the seat of a disorder appears in figure 4–1 on the next page.

Operating a Pendulum of Your Own

Anyone with a clear mind can learn to operate a pendulum. Here are some guidelines for picking one out and learning to work with it successfully.

Selecting a Pendulum

Many types of pendulums are available—exotic ones made of African wood and shaped like a bullet, sparkling crystals, steel or plastic varieties, ivory ones with a cavity for a witness, Lucite ones with needle points for the accurate reading of charts, and more. When selecting a pendulum for yourself, it is best to choose one that is clear, colorless, or of a neutral color such as gray, white, or black.

If you are a beginner, a fish line with a plumber's bob will work just fine. Make sure, however, that it is balanced and attached to a lightweight yet sturdy cord or chain. As you progress in radiesthesia, a more sensitive instrument might be in order. With experience, you will develop sensitivities that may heighten your appeal for a particular type of instrument. Selecting a pendulum, like choosing a ten-

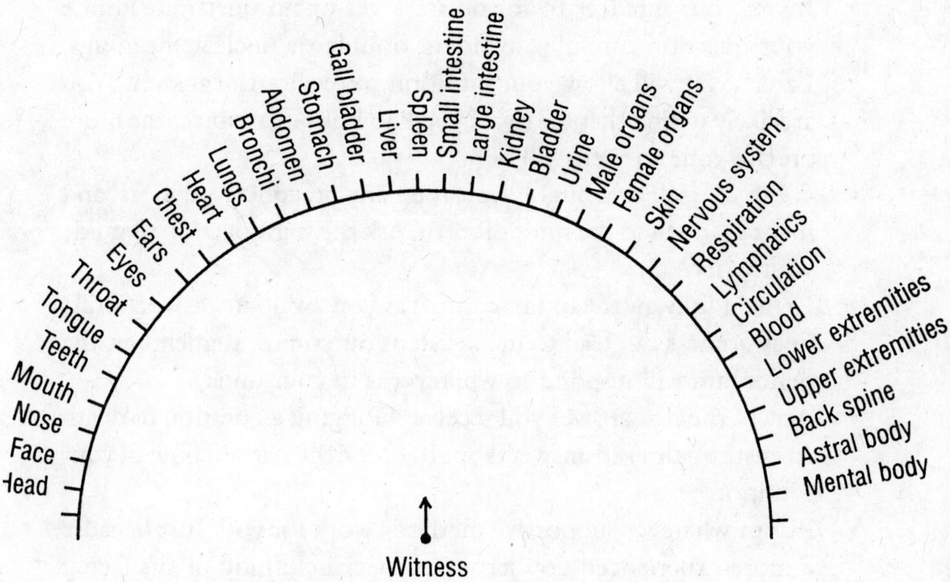

Figure 4–1 Seat of Disorder Chart

nis racquet, has a great deal to do with *feel*—so find the one that feels just right and use it consistently.

The pendulum, you will find, is only as good as its operator. Hence if you wish to do more than dabble with it, practice is essential. Why? Because with practice comes discernment. Dr. Aubrey T. Westlake of England once said that one of the most important functions of radiesthesia is to provide a bridge between two worlds—the sensible and the supersensible. "Learn to discriminate between the answers from the higher and lower selves," he added. "The difference is recognizable in [the higher self's] essential simplicity and truthful ring."

Rules to Dowse By

While working with your pendulum, observe the following rules. They will help you enhance your effectiveness as a dowser.

- Invite your intellect to formulate a yes-or-no question. Phrase your question carefully, avoiding double or unclear meanings. Later, you will allow your intuition to receive the answer. You are likely to find that the more you know about a subject the more precise your answers will be.
- Clear yourself thoroughly, releasing any preconceived ideas, and mentally open to the spirit of truth. Ask the spirit of truth to guide your work.
- Remain fully aware and in control as you await an answer. Shifts in awareness can lead to inconsistent outcomes. Remember, the pendulum will respond to whatever is in your mind.
- Accept the first answer you receive. Flogging a question to death to ensure a desired answer is apt to block the natural flow of your intuition.
- Adopt whatever supportive methods work for you. Just because a more experienced dowser wears special clothing or sits facing a certain direction to obtain correct answers, these practices may not be in your best interest. Find your *own* rituals and know that you are on the right path *for you.*
- Commit to using your pendulum only in your work. Avoid the temptation to use it for frivolities such as counting beans in a jar or seeking trivial information about your love life.

Tuning into Your Polarity

Another key to finding accurate answers with a pendulum lies in correctly interpreting its motion, which occurs in response to your polarity. Everything has polarity. These twin aspects of nature express themselves in such characteristics as yin-yang, feminine-masculine, dark-light, soft-hard, absorbing-deflecting, negative-positive, and so forth. Like the tides of magnetism, however, there is a point at which one polarity turns into its opposite, suggesting that there is no fixed yin or yang, for example; what was yin yesterday may be yang tomorrow.

A second aspect to keep in mind is that each of us, as we have learned, has a distinct pattern of radiatory energy—amounting to a composite of all the tissue building-blocks in our system. No matter how long we search, we will never find an exact duplicate of ourselves until we are perhaps able to produce a clone, and even then a precise replication may not be possible. In other words, the energy patterns you radiate while working with your pendulum cannot be matched by anyone else.

In addition to the composite polarity of an individual, each organ has its polarity, as does each cell and molecule. Dr. Albert Roy Davis and other magnetism researchers who have taken all these factors into account have found that the right side of the human body is often, though not always, positive (yes) and the left side negative (no).

The easiest way to find your yes-and-no reactions is to use a flashlight battery. Holding your pendulum between the thumb and index finger of your favored hand, suspend it from a length of string that allows for good swing over the positive (+) pole of the battery, and start the instrument moving a bit if you wish. Keeping your eyes focused on the pendulum, ask, "What is my positive reaction?" When the pendulum seems to be moving on its own, take note of its motion. Then change poles and proceed to find your negative reaction. Again take note of the motion you observe. Finally, alter the position of your fingers on the string until you have a length that allows for maximum action; the longer the string, the faster it goes. This entire procedure is called "tuning" your pendulum.

Between poles you will observe a third type of reaction—a more neutral motion. This action of the pendulum may indicate that something more is needed before you can obtain a definitive answer. When this occurs, you may have to clear yourself more thoroughly, reword your question, or even ask for preliminary information. Another possibility is that the information you are seeking is not available at this time. When in doubt about the meaning of a neutral motion, ask the pendulum!

The three basic actions of a pendulum are clockwise rotation, counterclockwise rotation, and oscillation to and fro. Variations on these motions are also common. What matters is not which motion reflects a yes or no response, but rather the *consistency* of that motion. After several trials, there should be no doubt in your mind that your positive reaction is, for example, a clockwise rotation.

Working with a Witness

The final component of dowsing for health is a witness—an item or bit of matter that carries the client's vibration. It is these definable radiations that will help you make a diagnostic evaluation or design a course of treatment. In the latter instance, you would test for resonance between the witness and a potential remedy. Ethically, of course, you would neither analyze nor evaluate treatments for a witness without the consent of the individual involved.

What might serve as a witness? One possibility is a photograph of the client. Many Aboriginal people disallow picture taking for fear that their souls will be "captured by the camera." And indeed a photograph of a person does hold a copy of their unique energy pattern and *aka* thread connections. For those who will allow it, and certainly for animals and plants, a photograph can convey a great deal about the subject both at the time the photograph was taken and in the present. As for the future, this can rarely be read with reliability.

Other suitable witnesses include sputum, urine, an original signature, a lock of hair, and a blood spot. Many well-established practitioners regard blood as the best possible witness. As Alice Bailey has stated in *Esoteric Psychology II,* "The blood is the life." This notion was expressed by Aart Jurriaanse when he wrote, in *Bridges,* "The blood system: this system centered in the heart is, in the first instance, the carrier of the life principle, and simultaneously also distributes the combined energies engendered or absorbed by the other bodily systems."

Although a blood spot may well be the most informative witness, please remember these two notes of caution. First, many practitioners today avoid the use of a blood witness because of the blood's capacity to transmit incurable diseases. Second, a practitioner of my acquaintance was using as a witness the blood of a hospitalized post-surgical client, when suddenly no reaction was registered over it. When the situation was checked out, it was found that the client had received a transfusion that had changed the characteristic life-energy code of her blood. It took more than twenty-four hours for the code to reassert itself, and only then was the practitioner able to get a reaction from the blood. The moral of this story is *readings from a blood spot may be impossible to get, or at the very least inaccurate, within twenty-four hours of a blood transfusion,* so plan on waiting it out while monitoring a client under these circumstances.

It is interesting to note that each blood cell carries the unmistakable energy blueprint of the individual from whom it originates. Energetically, this finding gives rise to many questions: What happens when cells from another pattern are superimposed onto an energy system? How long does it take for the individual to readjust? What happens during organ transplants or sex-change operations? Radiesthesia might someday spawn interesting answers to such questions.

Nobel Laureate Dr. Alexis Carrel advised physicians of the early twentieth century to keep their minds open to the possibility that unorthodox methods of medical investigation can be useful. Furthermore, he stated that radiesthesia is worthy of serious consideration.

In Europe and throughout much of the world, radiesthesia is indeed a science of the present as well as the past. In the United States, however, which can be amazingly innovative at some times and close-minded at others, radiesthesia is still considered a form of quackery. The good news is that with our population's increased recognition of energy patterns, dowsing for health is destined to become a viable research and treatment method here as well.

Chapter 5

Patterns

Interacting with the Subtle Bodies

> *The subject becomes aware of those basic patterns, forms and symbols which are the blueprints of the archetypes determining the evolutionary process, and which produce eventually the materializing of God's Plan. They are also the great symbols of man's unfolding consciousness. For instance, the recognition of the point, the line, the triangle, the square, the cross, the pentagon and similar symbols are simply the recognition of a connection with, and a founding upon, certain lines of force which have, to date, determined the evolutionary process.*
>
> —Alice A. Bailey

A pattern, or geometric design, is what makes something what it is. Look around and you will begin to notice a variety of basic shapes. These geometric configurations come from natural sources and act as links between natural forms. They also produce energy.

Many basic forms exist. An anthill has a triangular form △; the apex provides a small entry to a widening living area for the colony. A stalk of wheat or blade of grass has a vertical form. If you cut a cross section of a mint stem, you will find that it is square ❑.

The circle ○ may be the most important form of all. Among American Indian cultures, for instance, the circular medicine wheel has profound meaning. According to Hyemeyohsts Storm, author of *Seven Arrows:* "All things are contained within the Medicine Wheel, and all things are equal within it. The Medicine Wheel is the Total Universe." Storm further describes the medicine wheel as a mirror reflecting all that is.

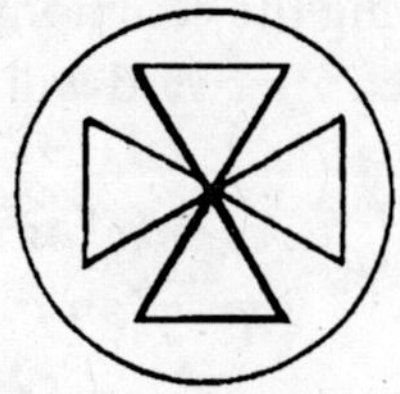

The circle circumscribes everything in the known world. Author and researcher Guenther Wachsmuth, in his study of etheric formative forces, suggested that the circle encloses all forces of nature and in the spectrum of light. The sixteenth-century alchemist and physician Paracelsus was even more specific when he wrote, "Everything that man accomplishes or does, that he teaches or wants to learn must have its right proportion; it must follow its own line and remain within its circle to the end that balance be preserved, that there be no crooked thing, that nothing exceed the circle."

With respect to circles as well as other configurations, a basic concept is that spirit moving outward from a vortex or center is *energy,* and energy streaming inward to a vortex or center becomes *matter,* as is demonstrated by the chakras. With this in mind, we can see that matter is an energy pattern. We might also imagine that, as Rudolf Steiner, early twentieth-century investigator of spiritual science, stated, etheric formative forces pour "centripetally inward from the circumference of cosmic space." When contained within a framed energy field, these inward-flowing forces are intensified—an important concept to remember while working with patterns.

The Curative Effect of Patterns

The use of patterns is as old as human history. Ancient petroglyphs contain numerous geometric configurations, such as the reverse swastika and circles, as well as figures of animals and symbols depicting the forces of nature, all of which may or may not have had medicinal value. We do know that contemporary Navajo singers (shamans) use geometrically decorated sand paintings in their curing ceremonies. Their symbolic patterns, ranging from simple to highly intricate, are designed in the moment to bring harmony and balance to a client. During the ceremony, the client will usually sit on the sand painting, which afterward will be destroyed.

> *A symbol as we know it is an outward and visible sign of an inward and spiritual reality.*
>
> —Alice A. Bailey

In the Middle Ages, alchemists and magicians alike used geometric forms. Some also chanted "sacred names"—what Hindus call *mantras*—combining sound with form energies. It has been noted that sound has a positive polarity whereas form has a negative one, and that together their polarity aspects give rise to color.

To experience the effects of such a practice, try meditating on the symbol of the heart chakra, shown below, while chanting its sound—"so-hum," which is Hindu for "He am I." "So," meaning "God," is expressed with the in-breath; "hum," meaning "I," is expressed on the out-breath. Typically, "so" is taken in through the left nostril and "hum" is exhaled through the right. When drawn out, the breaths produce the vibratory sound "soooooooo-hummmmmmmm." This *mantra* is known to help purify and calm the mind and feelings, since every breath taken in this way reminds us that we are part of God.

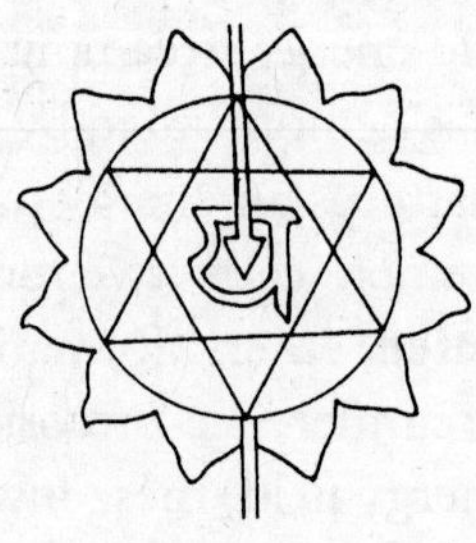

> *This may sound abstract to you, but sound is the "word" of consciousness by which form is built.*
>
> —Viola Petitt Neal, PhD

Other patterns to experiment with are the visually striking molecular structure symbols, such as that of germanium sesquioxide, shown in figure 5–1. Organic germanium, which greatly enriches the oxygen in the body, is found in such plants as ginseng, garlic, watercress, pearl barley, and comfrey.

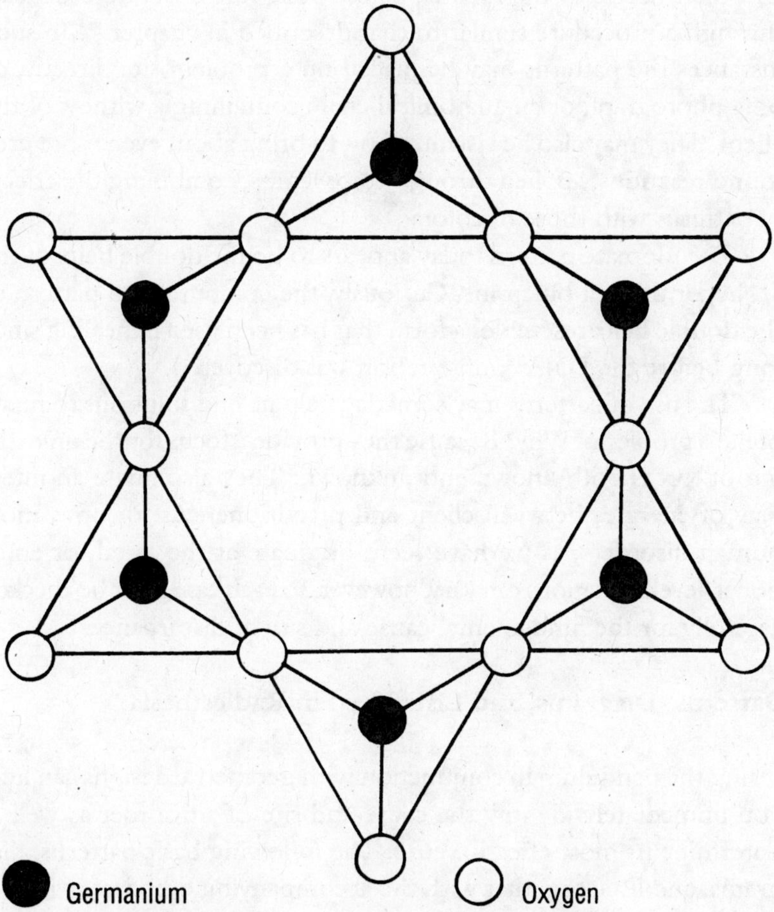

Figure 5–1 Molecular Pattern of Germanium Sesquioxide

Molecular symbols as well as other energy configurations are often used in radionic broadcasting, because they are known to profoundly affect the subtle bodies of the human energy system. As such, they are able to stimulate changes on the mental, astral, and physical/etheric levels. Dr. Aubrey T. Westlake's treatment patterns, as you will see in the next chapter, demonstrate this principle.

Many such correspondences are known. The circle, for instance, is said to be tuned to the astral body; the diamond shape to the etheric;

and the triangle to the mental. These basic forms can be broadcast through a procedure similar to that described in chapter 7. In such instances the patterns may be placed on a problem site directly, or on a photograph or an anatomical chart containing a witness of the client. They may also be visualized or, to bring about even more profound reactions, applied through color lamps, combining the effects of patterns with those of colors.

The ultimate pattern today appears to be the double helix of the DNA, or the cell blueprint. Curiously, the computerized pattern of the double helix resembles a form that has been used in healing since long before the DNA configuration was discovered.

The use of patterns may someday help us find solutions to many of life's problems. Why? Because they provide a focus for the unleashing of forces both known and unknown. They also invite an interplay of energies between client and practitioner. As for now, most human disorders, as we have seen, originate at the astral, or emotional, level. Situations can vary, however, so each case must be checked carefully for the fundamental cause and site of disturbance.

Patterns, Diagrams, and Lists Used in Radiesthesia

Using the pendulum in conjunction with geometric designs can help you immediately identify the cause and site of a disorder as well as determine its most effective cure. The following basic patterns, diagrams, and lists, together with the accompanying exercises, will give you a feel for the power of various configurations. The more you work with them, the more likely you are to develop modifications, and in the process personalize these tools for your own use.

Patterns

Patterns are most useful for broadcasting treatment. For one thing, they act as generators for sending particular energies to a witness; for another, they can be "set," like other radionic equipment, to transmit a desired frequency for a specified period of time. When broadcasting with a pattern it is vitally important to check the witness periodically, since your client's energies will change, as will his responses and needs.

Two of the more familiar patterns in use today are the Solomon Seal (also known as the Star of David) and the Static Diamond. Remember as you work with these configurations that the structure of any pattern creates waveforms and therefore specific energies.

Solomon Seal (Star of David). This configuration is frequently used in balancing. The type of waveform it generates seems to protect and shield one from the emotional impact of others. To experience its effects firsthand, try this exercise when you are about to engage in an emotionally trying encounter, such as an exam or a meeting with someone who irks you.

- Using a black marking pen, draw a Solomon seal ✡ on an 8½-by-11-inch sheet of white paper.
- Place your witness in the center of the symbol.
- Ask an assistant to remove your witness from the seal at a particular time during your encounter, and to replace it a few moments later.
- Embark on the encounter, checking your watch at the prearranged time. Did you feel different when the witness was removed?
- If not, try turning the seal in a different direction and repeating the experiment. Use the pendulum to guide you in finding the proper orientation.

Static Diamond. This treatment pattern is one of several developed by Dr. Aubrey Westlake and his colleagues in the mid-1970s. Their uses and methodologies are detailed in his book *The Pattern of Health,* where he refers to the static diamond as a "Jack of all trades."

Two of the major functions of this form are to energize Bach remedies or cell salts, which are described in chapter 9, and to help broadcast color therapy. When using it to energize a Bach remedy, the pattern should be oriented horizontally, as shown in figure 5–2, with the label for the cell salt Calcium sulphate facing north. Place the witness in the center of the diagram and the bottle containing the remedy on one of the circles marked "Bach." Then test the remedy with your pendulum to determine the correct dosage. In such instances the pendulum may also be used to find the correct remedy.

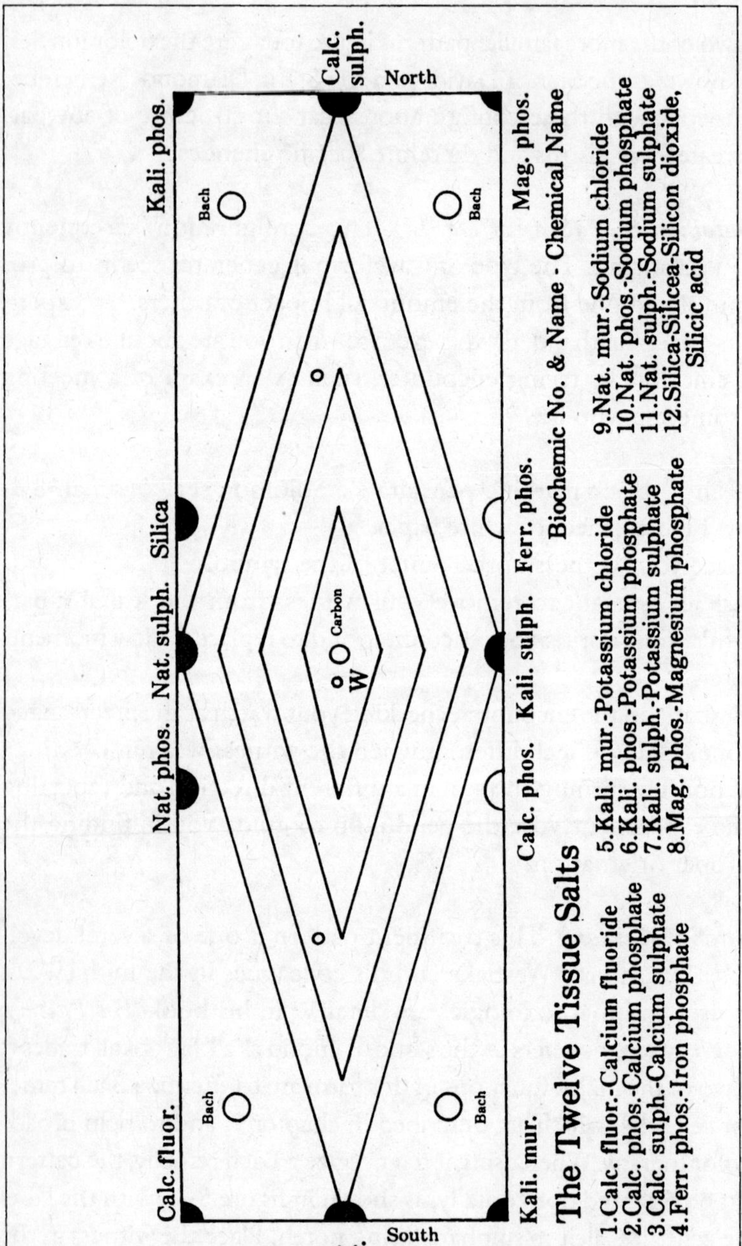

From *The Pattern of Health*, Aubrey Westlake, Shamballa, London, 1973
(Reproduced by permission of Mrs. Jean Westlake Cormack)

Figure 5–2 The Static Diamond

Diagrams

Geometrically designed diagrams are of great benefit to anyone dowsing for health. Each one has a place for the witness and spaces for writing the names of remedies, fruits, vegetables, grains, vitamins, or whatever potential cures the practitioner would like to test.

Following are two basic diagrams you can practice with. Feel free to devise your own variations on these themes or to compose original patterns if you prefer. The best guideline is: If it works for you, use it!

Wheel Diagram. Here the witness is placed at the hub, and items to be checked for compatibility are recorded at the ends of the twelve spokes. The pendulum, started over the witness, swings along a spoke to the proper item.

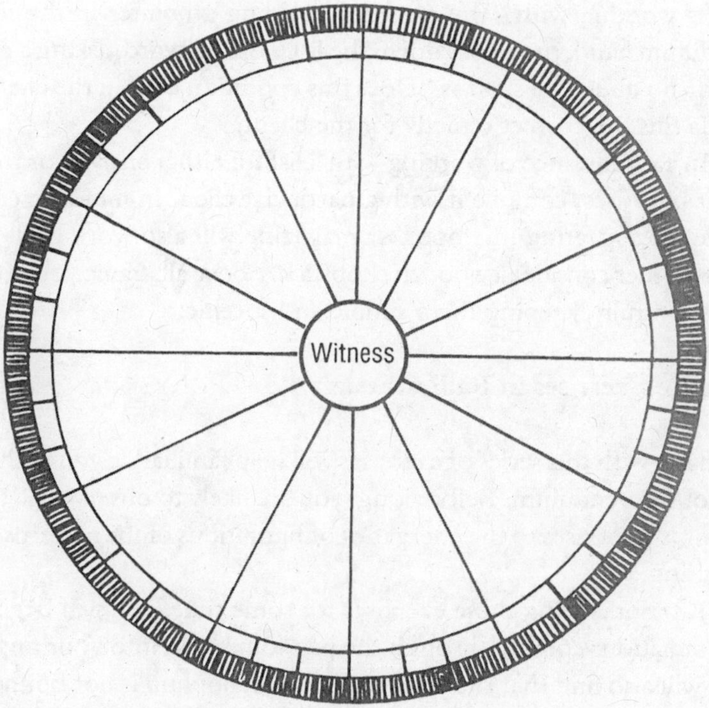

Figure 5–3 Wheel Diagram

V-Shaped Diagram. This diagram is extremely popular, perhaps because of its versatility. It may have only two lines—one for yes, another for no—or many lines labeled at the ends. The witness is placed at the apex (see figure 5–4), and the practitioner follows the same procedure as before until the pendulum points to the correct answer, the appropriate remedy, or as is illustrated here, the curative color.

Lists

Lists—simple vertical inventories—help radiesthesia practitioners assess the presence of dis-ease conditions, such as parasites. In addition they guide the practitioner to the needed remedial agent, such as a particular nutritional supplement, color, aromatherapy oil, gem therapy, flower essence, or whatever else is under consideration.

The list and the witness are usually placed on a sheet of black paper, since black is believed to deflect all radiations other than those one is working with. The operator, holding a pointer in the non-pendulum hand, then goes down the list word by word, asking a clear yes-or-no question, such as "Does this condition exist in the client?" or "Is this the correct remedy for the client?"

In each instance of working with a list for either analytic or treatment purposes, compile it with a particular client in mind; a ready-made list appearing in a book or magazine will also work well. For your pointer consider a wooden chopstick. Above all, frame your questions carefully, keeping them simple and specific.

Practice Exercises in Radiesthesia

Working with this series of exercises will help familiarize you with the feel of the pendulum. Before long, you are likely to observe the pendulum's responses to the energetic configurations of the patterns you are using.

After practicing these exercises for some time, you will begin to feel radiations coming through the pendulum and into your fingers. You will also find that the activity of your pendulum is not bound by forces operating on the physical plane.

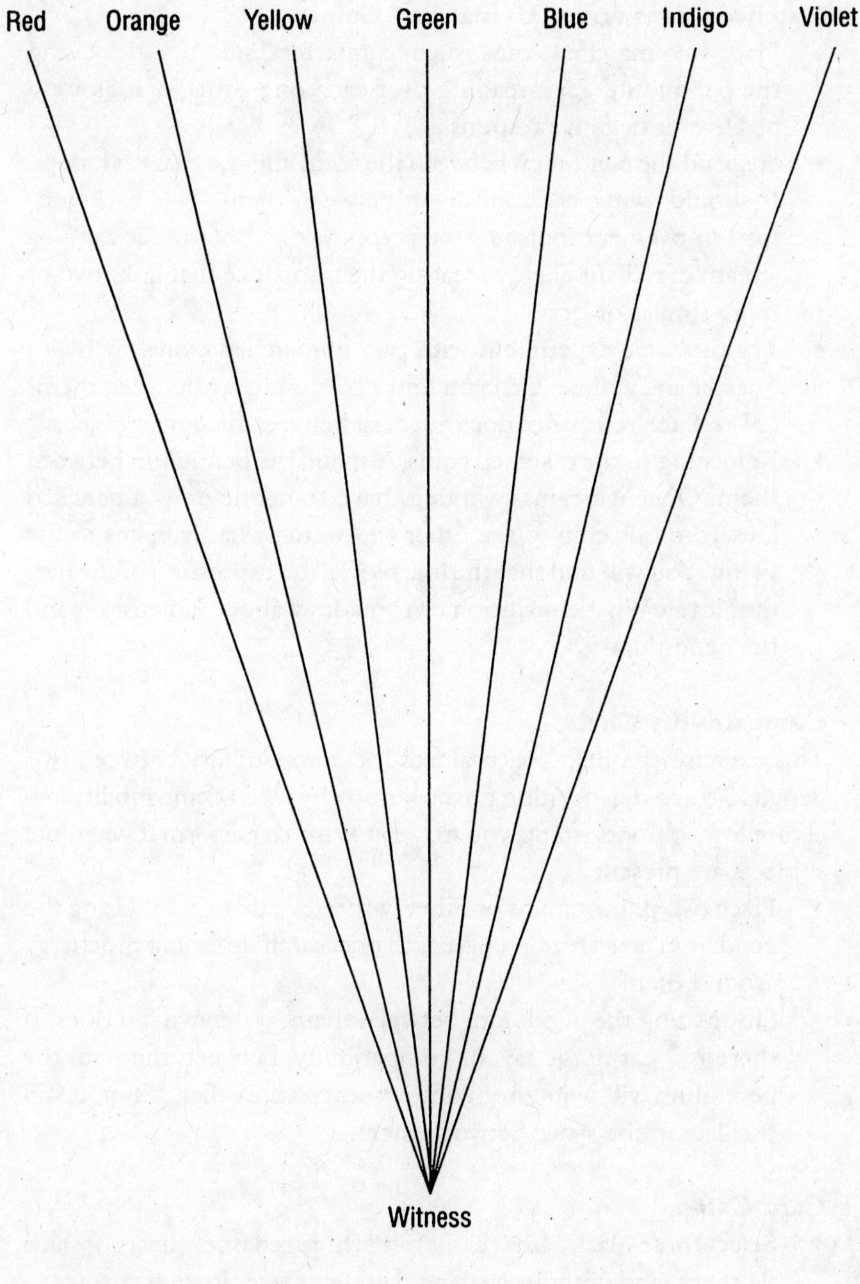

Figure 5–4 V-Shaped Diagram

Matched Coins versus Unmatched Coins

- Place two matched coins, such as quarters, side by side. Using the pendulum, get a reading over each one—that is, look for a positive or negative response.
- Suspend the pendulum between the coins and watch what it does. It should swing back and forth between them. This back-and-forth movement indicates the presence of a "harmonic ray"—a stream of radiant energy creating the resonance that links two or more similar objects.
- Try the same experiment with two *un*matched coins, such as a quarter and a dime. Can you find a harmonic ray between them? (*Note:* Such resonance does not exist between dissimilar objects!)
- Returning to the matched coins, suspend the pendulum between them. Once it begins swinging, have someone draw a penciled line from one coin to the other and watch what happens to the swing. You will find that the line blocks the expression of the harmonic ray. What conclusion can you draw about dimensions and the pendulum?

Compatibility Check

This exercise can help you evaluate the compatibility between two people. To avoid generating further antipathy when compatibility levels are low or nonexistent, you may *not* want to perform it when the subjects are present.

- Place two photographs or other witnesses side by side. Using the pendulum, get a reading over each one, carefully feeling the energy around them.
- Suspending the pendulum between them, watch what it does. If there is a harmonic ray, or compatibility, between the two, the pendulum will swing from one witness to the other. If not, it will oscillate in the space between them.

Card Game

- Select three black cards (clubs) and three red ones (hearts), shuffle them, and without looking, lay them face down in a row.
- Mentally program your pendulum to do a negative swing over the black cards and a positive swing over the red ones.

- Setting the pendulum over the card farthest to the left, observe the swing, turn over the card, and give yourself one point for an accurate reading.
- Repeat the previous step with each of the five remaining cards. How successful were you at programming your pendulum?

Guess the Thought Form (an advanced group practice)
- Divide a group of people into two teams, A and B.
- Ask one member of team B to leave the room while team A builds a thought form on a table. (To build a thought form, one simply thinks of an object, such as a Ping-Pong ball, concentrating on its shape.)
- Invite the team B member back into the room to dowse the shape on the table while asking yes-or-no questions of her teammates. When she guesses the thought form, she scores one point for her team. If a specified period of time goes by without a correct guess, go to the next step.
- Repeat this exercise with team B building a thought form and a team A member dowsing for the answer.
- Continue alternating between builders and dowsers, scoring one point for each correct guess. Then give a prize to the team that scores the most points.

Hand Analysis
- Hold your pendulum over each portion of the hand analysis chart shown in figure 5–5 and ask, "Is this area balanced?" The answers you get should tell you a good deal about your physical well-being and areas in need of balance.
- Repeat this exercise using a witness and, if you wish, a pointer. The witness may be placed on various portions of the hand shown on the chart, and then tested in each location. Or you could set it beside the illustrated hand and, using a pointer, conduct the test over the witness. Enjoy and have fun!

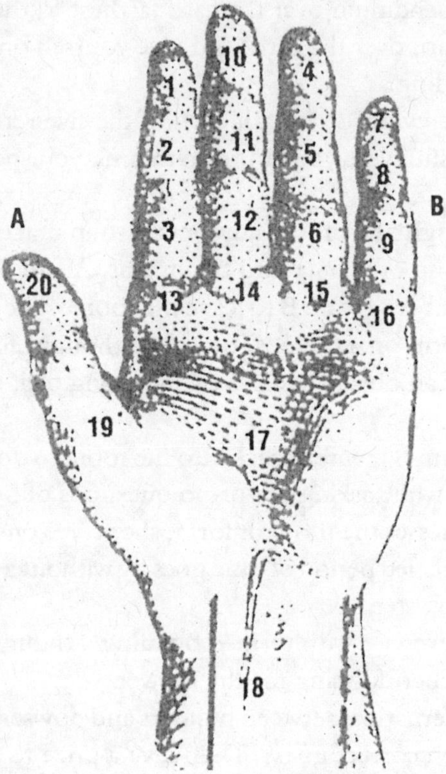

1. Head
2. Throat
3. Arms, hands, shoulders
4. Chest
5. Stomach
6. Intestines
7. Kidneys, spine
8. Sex organs
9. Thighs, anus
10. Knees
11. Legs
12. Feet
13. Liver, circulation
14. Bones, teeth
15. Heart
16. Nervous system
17. Facial muscles
18. Abdominal muscles, chest muscles
19. Throat muscles
20. General vitality

A, B—Areas in which variations occur during menstruation in women and about seven times a year in males

Figure 5–5 Hand Analysis Chart

Chapter 6

Healing at a Distance

Mind As a Generator

The force of mind. This is the illuminating energy which lights the way of an idea or form to be transmitted and received. Forget not that light is a subtle substance. Upon a beam of light can the energy of mind materialize.

—Alice A. Bailey

The therapeutic art of radionics, or healing at a distance, transcends the ordinary parameters of scientific explanation. Its applications are limitless, bounded only by the creative abilities and skills of practitioners, and its therapeutic effects are often profound. Why? Most likely because radionics is based on universal laws. It recognizes that each person, a unique combination of substance and essence, is imbued with both material and subtle components. Moreover, it acknowledges the universality of consciousness—that we are part of everything that exists. Ultimately, radionics serves as a bridge not only between physical and nonphysical realities but between orthodox and spiritual medicine.

British practitioner Mrs. Lavender Dower, MRadA, who has worked in radionics for more than half a century, sees it as the medicine of the future, especially now that science is catching on to the concept of energy medicine and the existence of chakras. In answer to the question "How does radionics achieve its results?" she says: "I am discovering new things every day, and I believe that communication may be the key to how radionics works. Energy and conscious intelligence appear to be linked down to a cellular level, and reawakening the integrity of the structure at fault, at any level, may explain what we are doing."

Mrs. Dower, like most practitioners, believes that the success of radionics depends on the powers of the practitioner which, interestingly enough, have little to do with proximity to the client and everything to do with the unique capacities of the human mind. Indeed, radionics distinguishes itself from other analysis and treatment practices by its ability to bring about healing at a distance.

A Brief History of Healing at a Distance

Radionic techniques, first developed by two Californians, has had a dismal history in the United States. Albert Abrams, AM, LLD, MD, ignited the spark of radionics in the first decade of the twentieth century. Often called the father of radionics, this highly respected physician was director of clinical medicine at Leland Stanford University. His research, which he personally financed, revealed, among other things, that certain substances appeared to neutralize particular diseases—more specifically, that radiations of these substances counterbalanced radiations of the diseases. Using a black wooden box, he was also able to detect diseases before physical symptoms manifested. As such, he was the first person to practice analysis at a distance, with no visible or tangible link between himself and the client. The intriguing story of Dr. Abrams's work is documented in his book *New Concepts in Disease and Diagnosis* (listed in the resource section at the back of this book).

Dr. Ruth Drown, a chiropractor in the late 1920s, was the second practitioner to pioneer openly in the field of radionics. Having worked for Abrams earlier in that decade, Dr. Drown had learned his methods and used his instruments, which by then were available around the world. She went on to develop instruments of her own and, like Abrams, to experience great success in healing. By then she had many cancer cures to her credit, which may have led to her persecution. After an apparently trumped-up trial, she was convicted of fraud and jailed.

A contemporary noted that "she was in touch with a tremendously complicated internal system of patterned harmonics, a self-regulating system of resonant vibrations," and attributed her demise to the fact that she was the first person to develop and apply distant therapy, which she called "radio therapy." Working with a patient's witness, she had no need to see the person face-to-face. In addition, she was the first to recognize the importance of treating the endocrine glands and to do radionic photography. Convinced that a person's body energy provided the only current needed for analysis, remedy selection, and treatment, she used no commercial electricity to operate her instruments.

As a result, no doubt, of the powerful and oftentimes closed medical system in place in the United States, the radionic torch moved overseas to England. There George delaWarr, an engineer and inventive genius, expanded on this dynamic discipline together with his wife, Marjorie, at their laboratory in Oxford. Another Englishman, David V. Tansley, followed up with studies on the influence of cosmic ray energies, addressed in chapter 10.

The stories of Abrams, Drown, delaWarr, Tansley, and other British pioneers such as Guyon Richards, MD, and Malcolm Rae, inventor of the Rae system, are well documented in several of the volumes listed at the back of this book. An excellent account of radionics' stormy and fascinating history in agriculture as well as in healing can be found in *Report on Radionics* by Edward W. Russell.

Today, England continues to sanction radionics. Considerable research in this science is also taking place in Russia and India. In the United States, still subject to political pressures from the American Medical Association and a burgeoning drug industry, radionic research and practice continue, but in a much more guarded manner than in other parts of the world.

The Powers of Mind

The single most important characteristic of radionic practice is the exercise of divinely inspired mental powers that are ours by birthright. All of us have this capacity, although in most individuals it remains hidden, unused, or even more regrettably, unacknowledged. In fact, it is mind that enables radionic practitioners to treat at a distance. In *A Treatise on White Magic,* Alice Bailey explains how these healing energies can be utilized: "The need for realizing that the etheric body is vitalized and controlled by thought can be brought into full functioning activity. The [practitioner] breathes deeply, he concentrates his mind and drives the thought from him."

Once a client signals an *intent* for help, the practitioner engages thought to establish an energy connection through which healing forces may be directed. This pattern of contact is sometimes represented by a triangle showing at its base the practitioner and client in physical form across a vast distance, and at its apex the point in another dimension where the healing takes place, often immediately upon "contact" between the two.

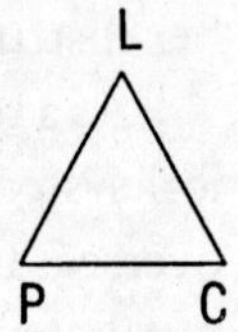

This aspect of radionic practice is explained, as follows, on the back cover of the time-honored British Radionic Association's *Radionic Journal:* "[Radionics] is a method of healing at a distance through the medium of an instrument using the ESP faculty. In this way, a trained and competent practitioner can discover the cause of disease within any living system, be it a human being, an animal, a plant, or the soil itself. Suitable therapeutic energies can then be made available to the patient to help restore optimum health."

What exactly *is* this condition we call disease? In the words of the late George Starr-White, MD, of California, whose books were at least fifty years ahead of their time: "Contrary to popular belief, and although we place names on given ailments, there is only one state of disease and one state of health. There is a great variation between the two, and if we live *with* nature instead of *for* nature then we may to some extent overcome these diseases."

Research informs us that all living things are composed of light and vibration. When something interferes with the rhythmic vibrational rate of an organism, the consequences are felt within it. This dissonance, of one type or another, is what we call "disease." Navajo people call it "disharmony"—a far more accurate term!

We are only now beginning to understand what Native American healers have known for centuries—that harmony is largely dependent on thought. Thought, in other words, plays a key role in wellness. Visualization work conducted by such mid-twentieth-century healers as O. Carl and Stephanie Simonton, as well as Shakti Gawain, have for years been demonstrating the power of thought. Their conclusion is, *we are what we think!* Indeed, the universe itself, according to the eminent British scientist Sir James Jeans, is "like a great thought." So, too, are we—and perhaps a holographic one at that!

> *Do not believe that health is retained or maintained through doctors; nor can drugs guarantee it. If that were the case, then all the dead should be alive now.*
>
> —Sri Sathya Sai Baba

The etheric body is where radionic practitioners focus much of their attention and thought. By directing their attention to this subtle body, they are able to detect disharmony, and through the power of thought, they can succeed in treating it—all before it manifests on the gross physical level. If such an approach were widely practiced, what a boon this could be to humanity!

Supportive Equipment

The mind as a generator allows radionic practitioners to engage in a thought-energized form of analysis and consequent treatment. Most make use of analysis forms and instruments as vehicles for focusing their thought. All such vehicles can, in the hands of a gifted practitioner, be used creatively and effectively. Here we will begin by looking at instruments used for analysis and treatment; then we'll explore forms commonly employed for analysis.

Instruments

The basic radionic instrument is a variation on Albert Abrams's black wooden box. It allows practitioners to pinpoint their focus and hold the thought through the setting on a potency dial. In a sense, the instrument *defines* the thought it is to measure, serving as a quality control mechanism for a particular treatment that can then be duplicated. Setting the dial to a vibratory rate enables the practitioner to maintain a particular focus for the duration of the treatment—a task impossible to accomplish with only our "monkey minds."

To augment the effectiveness of thought-energized treatment, Englishman Malcolm Rae, in the 1960s, developed a box with a card slot, known as a Mark III instrument (see figure 6–2), together with a series of treatment cards based on the underlying geometric patterns of a multitude of phenomena from a particular bacteria to an emotional state, such as love (see figure 6–1). Rae cards are in widespread use among present-day radionic practitioners. The relevant card, in conjunction with the appropriate vibratory rate of thought, establishes the treatment to be broadcast. Whereas the rate setting sustains projection of a thought wave, the geometrical pattern appears to tune its energy.

Analysis Forms

To assess disharmony in the etheric body, radionic practitioners conduct an analysis, measuring the degree of deviation between a perfect condition and the imperfect one exhibited by the witness placed on or near the form. Any time a deviation is found, it is evaluated numerically.

The British analysis forms shown in figures 6–3 and 6–4 reveal two different systems of measurement. Both call for dowsing, to achieve an accurate reading of the etheric body's energy waves. Both also assist in arriving at a meaningful graph that provides an overall "picture" of the condition. Individual details can then be evaluated.

An analysis form conceived by Dr. Hazel Parcells, of New Mexico, is based on a scale of 360 as a perfect functional reading—reflecting a balance of all elements needed for life energy—and of 120 as a functional norm, or sustaining level, in other areas (see figure 6–5). Each

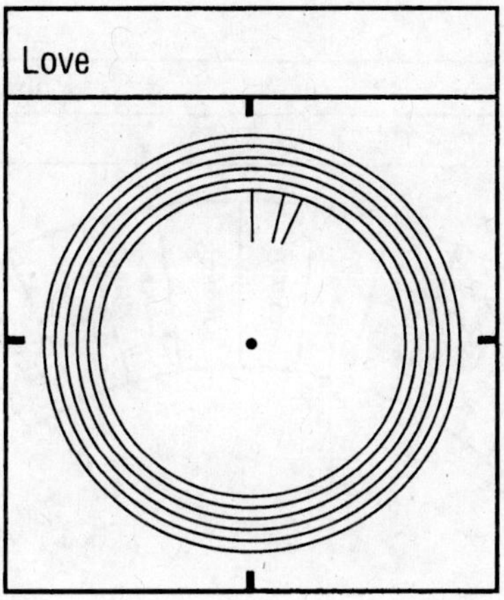

Figure 6–1 Rae Card

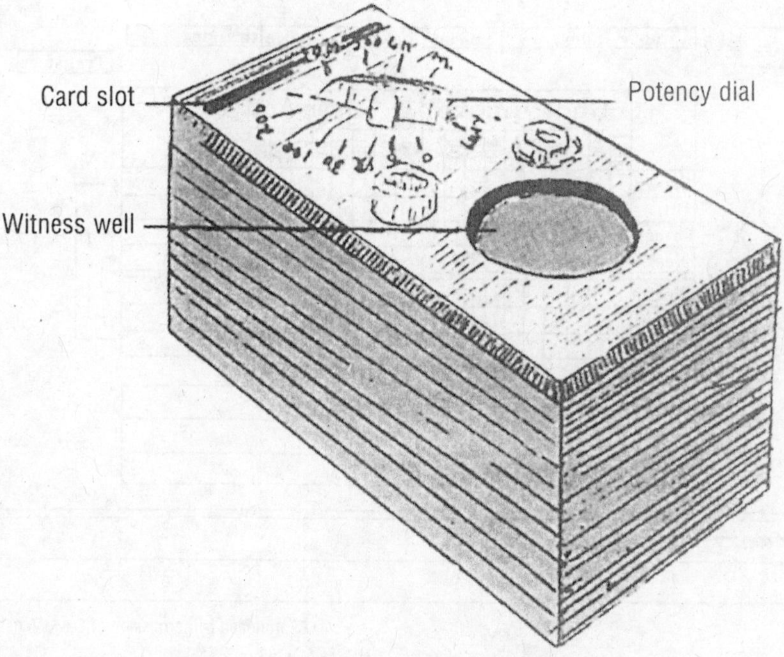

Figure 6–2 Mark III Instrument

Name: **Age:** **Date:**

Address: **Phone:**

Symptoms:

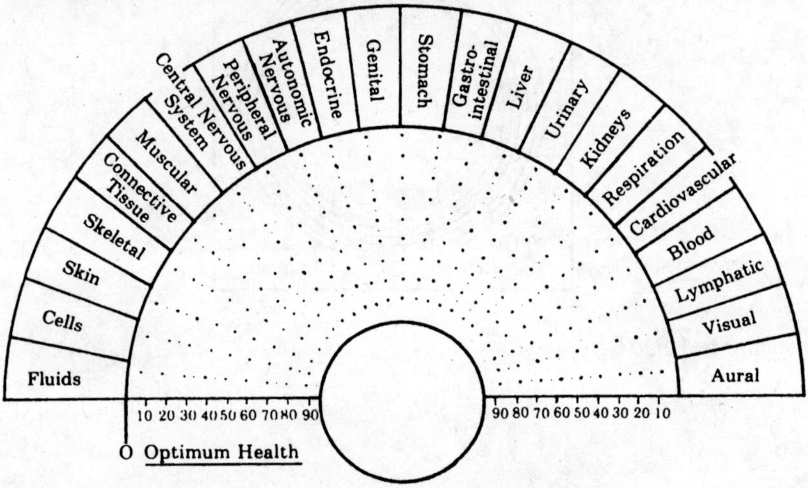

Rays

Vitality Index:	Spleen Chakra:	Health Index:

Transfers

	Under-Active										Normal	Over-Active										
	100	90	80	70	60	50	40	30	20	10		10	20	30	40	50	60	70	80	90	100	
Crown																						
Brow																						
Throat																						
Heart																						
Solar Plexus																						
Sacral																						
Base																						

Congestion:	Miasms:
Over-Stimulation:	Toxins:
Lack of Co-Ordination:	

Primary Treatment:

Reproduced by permission of David Tansley

Figure 6–3 Analysis Form (British)

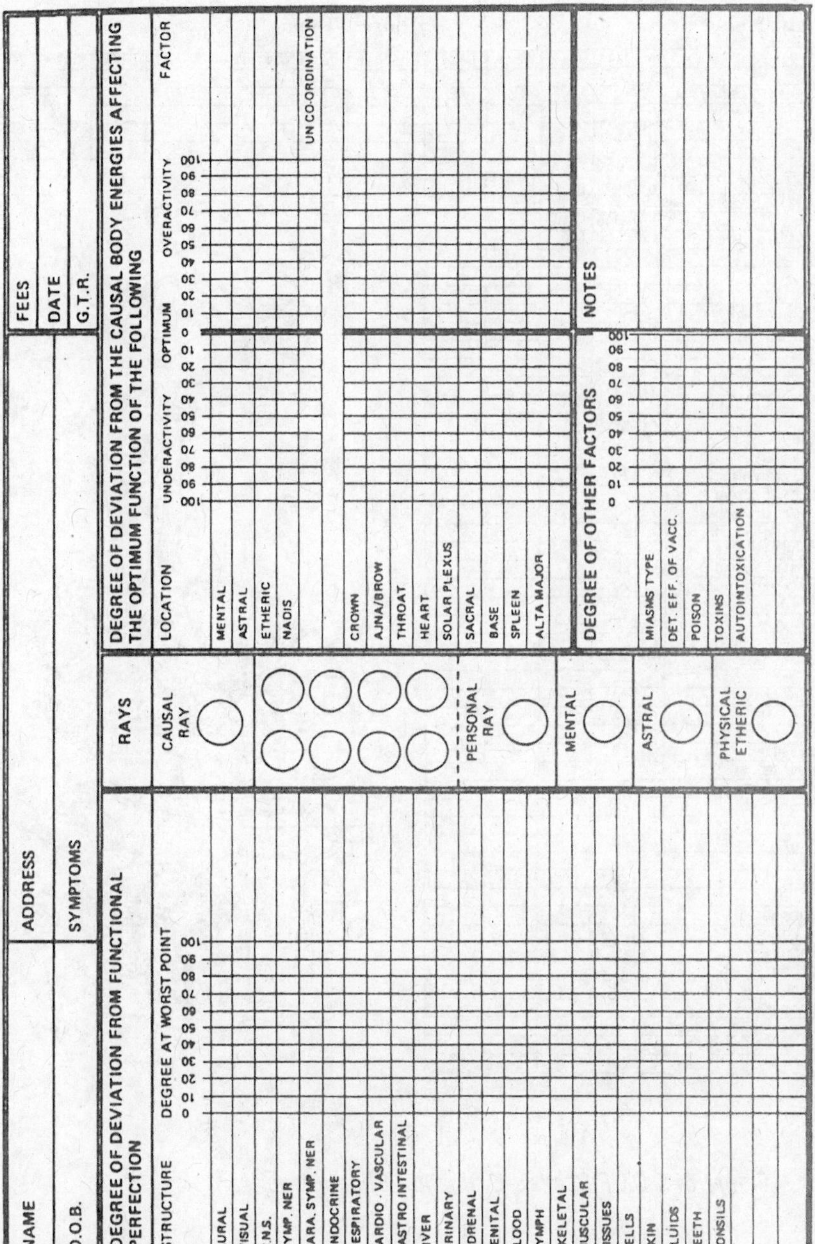

NAME

D.O.B.

ADDRESS

SYMPTOMS

FEES

DATE

G.T.R.

DEGREE OF DEVIATION FROM FUNCTIONAL PERFECTION

STRUCTURE

DEGREE AT WORST POINT

0 10 20 30 40 50 60 70 80 90 100

AURAL

VISUAL

C.N.S.

SYMP. NER

PARA. SYMP. NER

ENDOCRINE

RESPIRATORY

CARDIO . VASCULAR

GASTRO INTESTINAL

LIVER

URINARY

ADRENAL

GENITAL

BLOOD

LYMPH

SKELETAL

MUSCULAR

TISSUES

CELLS

SKIN

FLUIDS

TEETH

TONSILS

RAYS

CAUSAL RAY

PERSONAL RAY

MENTAL

ASTRAL

PHYSICAL ETHERIC

DEGREE OF DEVIATION FROM THE CAUSAL BODY ENERGIES AFFECTING THE OPTIMUM FUNCTION OF THE FOLLOWING

LOCATION

UNDERACTIVITY

100 90 80 70 60 50 40 30 20 10

OPTIMUM

0

OVERACTIVITY

10 20 30 40 50 60 70 80 90 100

FACTOR

MENTAL

ASTRAL

ETHERIC

NADIS

UN CO-ORDINATION

CROWN

AJNA/BROW

THROAT

HEART

SOLAR PLEXUS

SACRAL

BASE

SPLEEN

ALTA MAJOR

DEGREE OF OTHER FACTORS

0 10 20 30 40 50 60 70 80 90 100

NOTES

MIASMS TYPE

DET. EFF. OF VACC.

POISON

TOXINS

AUTOINTOXICATION

Reproduced by permission of Magneto Geometric Applications

Figure 6–4 Subtle Anatomy Analysis Form (British)

Patient Name Address/Phone

	Normals	Date	Date	Date
A/A				
Physical Energy				
Etheric Energy				
Blood Sugar	80-120			
Total Lipids	450-500			
Fatty Acids	190-450			
Cholesterol	130-230			
Calcium	9.5-11.0			
Sodium	310-345			
Sod. Chloride	450-500			
Potassium	16-22			
Magnesium	1-3			
Phos. Inorgan.	3.7-5			
Red Blood Energy	140			
White Blood Energy	135			
Hemoglobin	80-95			
Total Proteins	6.5-8.2			
Albumin	3.0-3.7			
Total Nitrogen	3.0-3.7			
Uric Acid	2.0-3.5			
GLANDS				
Pineal Gland	120			
Pituitary Whole	120			
Anterior Lobe	120			
Posterior Lobe	120			
Parotid Gland	120			
Lymphatic Organs	120			
Thyroid Gland	120			
Parathyroid Gland	120			
Spleen	120			
Thymus	120			
Ovaries	120			
Ova Testae	120			
Stilbesterol	120			
Testosterone	120			
Orcitinum	120			
Progesterone	120			
Prostate	120			
Placenta	120			
Corpus Luteum	120			
Suprarenal	120			
Adrenal Cortex	120			
Adrenal Medulla	120			
LUNGS				
Int. Lobe - L.	120			
Int. Lobe - R.	120			
Mid Lobe - L.	120			
Mid Lobe - R.	120			
Bronchus - L.	120			
Bronchus - R.	120			
Bronchus - Total	120			
Pulmonary Artery	120			
L. Br. Pulm. Art.	120			
R. Br. Pulm. Art.	120			
L. U&L Pulm. Vein	120			

1.08

No. Date	Date	Date	Cultures	Date	Date	Date
1						
2						
3						
4						
5						
6						
7						

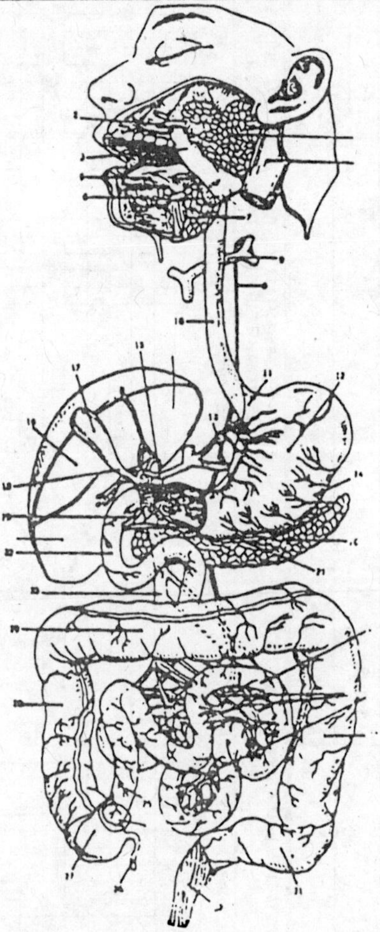

Figure 6–5 Dr. Parcells's Evaluation Sheet (American)

Notes

KIDNEY

1 ____ Capsule
2 ____ Cortex
3 ____ Pyramids
4 ____ Renal Tubules
5 ____ Malpighian
6 ____ Renal Papillae
7 ____ Medulla
8 ____ Pelvis
9 ____ Ureter
10 ____ Renal Vein
11 ____ Renal Artery
12 ____ Hilus
13 ____ Calyx

URINARY BLADDER & KIDNEYS

10 ____ Urethral Orifice
11 ____ Urethra
12 ____ Opening of Ureter
13 ____ Urinary Bladder
14 ____ Ureter

FEMALE PELVIC ORGANS

7 ____ Fallopian Tube
8 ____ Fundus of Uterus
9 ____ Uterine Wall
10 ____ Cervix of Uterus
11 ____ Vagina
19 ____ Fallopian Tube
20 ____ Masovarium
21 ____ Ovary - Right
22 ____ Ovary - Left
23 ____ Fimbrae of Uterine Tube

MALE PELVIC ORGANS

7 ____ Scrotum
8 ____ Inner Intequment of Testes
9 ____ Testicle
14 ____ Glans Penis
15 ____ Urethra
16 ____ Bulbo-Cavernosus Muscle
17 ____ Corpus Cavernosum Urethrae
18 ____ Cowper's Gland
19 ____ Corpus Cavernosum Penis
20 ____ Urogenital Diaphragm
21 ____ Prostate Gland
23 ____ Deferent Duct
24 ____ Ureteral Orifice in Bladder
26 ____ Apex of Urinary Bladder
27 ____ Deferent Duct Entering

____ Venous Circulation
____ Arterial Circulation

DATE	BROADCASTS

Reproduced by permission of Dr. Hazel R. Parcells

reading is evaluated in relation to others on the form. Ultimately, mathematical scales are the best way to analyze a client's situation, both for accurate baseline assessments and for future comparisons.

In addition to assessing the condition of the etheric body, radionic practitioners are able to examine, through dowsing, conditions of the personality that appear in the physical, astral, and mental bodies. Beyond that, we do not seem to have the capacity of consciousness to investigate. We may try, as humans typically do, but our reliability would be subject to question. Why? Because beyond the personality, we are dealing with the spiritual nature which, in its infinite wisdom and detachment, most likely tolerates yet defies much that we do in our basic "earth school"!

Conducting a Practice Analysis

Try this practice analysis to familiarize yourself with some of the principles involved in working at a distance. Once you are comfortable with the process, you will be able to pay more attention to the vibratory subtleties you are working with.

Each step of the way, you will be following the analysis form of your choice and using radiesthesia to find answers. Analyzing at a distance, you will note, is different from treating at a distance. Whereas treatment makes use of a radionic instrument, analyzing through radiesthesia requires you to use your *body* as the instrument.

Practice often—with yourself, friends, family members, and pets. The more experience you acquire in radionic analysis, the greater your understanding will be and the more techniques you will develop on your own.

Materials

To perform a practice analysis you will need a quiet space in which to work, along with the following items:

- An analysis form, together with a chart or diagrams of the anatomy, lists of remedies and disorders, and radiesthetic scales
- A pendulum
- A notebook on which to place materials

- A witness or other materials you wish to test. The witness, as described in chapter 4, can be a blood spot or, preferably, a photograph, a lock of hair, sputum, urine, or an original signature. It should be plainly marked in pencil with the person's name and the date. A "word witness" may also be used, provided that permission has been granted; for this you would pencil in the person's name in block letters on a sheet of white paper.
- A clear and open mind
- *Optional:* Black paper to cover your work space and a small magnet for clearing the space

Procedure

- Lay out the form, chart, and materials. (A work space covered with black paper is believed to pose a barrier to all radiations other than those you are analyzing.) Then center and thoroughly clear yourself.
- Place the witness in your work space—or better yet, on the chart, if a place for the witness is provided.
- Working with your pendulum and the chart, pose questions carefully and clearly. For example, if you are using the chart illustrated in figure 6–4, you might ask: "Is the aural reading balanced (functionally perfect)?" If the answer is no, ask for the degree of deviation—10? 20? 30? Record on the chart each finding as you get it, then move on to the next area of investigation.
- Once you have proceeded to the subtle body readings, you might ask, for example: "Is the mental body functioning optimally?" If the answer is no, ask, "Is it underactive?" "Overactive?" Then ask for the degree of deviation—10? 20? 30? Record your findings and continue on to the next subtle body reading.

Going Further

- Look for relationships between the various chakra functions and effects that may be showing up in the corresponding organs. In each instance, be sure to ask for the *fundamental state* of each chakra. If you don't, your readings may be tempered by more superficial energies transmitted by moods, environmental forces, or even the phase of the moon.

- Ascertain the rays that reflect how the person functions, and note their effects on the physical organism. (See chapter 10 for information on the seven rays.)
- Check for the presence of a ***miasm***—defined by George Vithoulkas, MIH, in *The Science of Homeopathy,* as "a predisposition towards chronic disease underlying the acute manifestation of illness, (1) which is transmissible from one generation to another, and (2) which may respond beneficially to the corresponding nosode [remedy] prepared either from pathological tissue or from the appropriate drug or vaccine."

  The esoteric explanation for a miasm is this: when we incarnate, we take some of the earth's etheric energy to form our own etheric vehicle, which may then become contaminated by the tuberculosis, cancer, syphilis, or other illnesses once suffered by uncountable numbers of diseased people buried underground. In other words, the taint of disease remains within the etheric body of the earth and may show up, anytime after a person's birth, as a predisposition toward that illness.

  Chronic conditions that do not respond to treatment are frequently related to miasms. Hence, good detective work at the outset can have predictive value as time passes. As David Tansley said, "Greater success in radionic assessments can be achieved with a foreknowledge f the homeopathic principles of miasms."
- Be on the lookout for congestion, overstimulation, and lack of coordination, each of which may indicate a chakra that is out of balance.
- Pinpoint specific environmental poisons and toxins that may be affecting the person. Be sure to check for mercury amalgam fillings, as well as other metallics such as aluminum and lead. Knowing the culprit is step one in finding the neutralizing radiations.

The Future of Healing at a Distance

Considering all that we know of energy systems and the forces governing human well-being, it seems that for true healing to take place, a client must on some level participate in their own treatment. Other than physical adjustments such as skeletal manipulation and surgical procedures, there appear to be only two ways to encourage a client to correct an imbalance. One is by providing the on-site energy needed to remedy the disorder by, for example, applying electrical stimulation for fracture repair, or other forms of electromagnetic therapy. The second way to bring about change is to give the client *coded instructions for self-generated healing*.

Such coded instructions are the domain of radionics, and they are introduced by transmitting subtle force-field vibratory rates of well-being from afar. These energies—projected via Rae cards or dialed rates, or both—modify not only imbalances but also the encoding that gave rise to them, "reminding" the client of their inherent capacity to live in harmony.

The art of healing at a distance, despite all the progress and success it has seen since the days of Albert Abrams and Ruth Drown, is still not explainable by the scientific method. Consequently, it may never be "legitimized" enough to satisfy the scientific and medical communities. More than likely, it will march to its own drummer, *cooperating with* mainstream health professions yet never *becoming* one. Its unique blend of scientific and esoteric knowledge will keep it "not quite empirical" and at the same time effectively authentic—which may be for the best. We are, after all, complex beings bonded to worlds beyond our comprehension. And radionics, together with its complement radiesthesia, provides a means for reaching into these realms and accessing the extraordinary information they hold for us.

Chapter 7

Broadcasting Techniques

Projecting Healing Vibrations

Then by an act of will, resulting in a breathing forth, and engendered or arrived at dynamically in the interlude of contemplation or retention of breath, the created form is sent forth into the phenomenal world...

—Alice A. Bailey

The driving force behind radionics is broadcasting—the means by which thought forms are focused, energized, and sent on a path to their target. Broadcasting requires breath control and the ability to formulate thought forms, or patterns of projections. The operator, in other words, must be capable of concentration and single-pointed thought, capacities that are best developed through the practice of meditation.

Of the meditation methods known to Westerners, perhaps the simplest and most effective one for focusing is the candle-gazing technique recommended by Sri Sathya Sai Baba, an acknowledged Avatar—Sanskrit for "one who descends." Here a person concentrates on the flame of a candle, pinpointing the mind exclusively on the light. Instructions for this technique are spelled out in the appendix on page 133. *Pranayama,* the yogic discipline of breathing, also helps us focus energy on patterns that are being projected. Typical patterns for broadcasting include the Solomon Seal or Static Diamond illustrated in chapter 5, the Magnetron design shown on page 66, or representations of molecular structures, each with its own waveform configuration.

Assisting the mind in projecting healing vibrations are numerous radionic instruments. Their costs vary, depending on the circuitry involved. Whereas some instruments are quite simple, others offer an array of sophisticated gadgetry such as blinking lights, fancy keyboards, and digital readouts.

> *By the use of an instrument, the thought may be stabilized for any length of time.*
>
> —Malcolm Rae

The material that follows explores a variety of broadcasting techniques. After trying some of them, you may feel a desire to develop methods of your own. If you do, by all means experiment, practice, and freely use whatever works for *you*. All the while, be sure to keep records so that before moving on, you will know the factors that have been most effective. Also keep in mind the fact that all clients—whether they are people, pets, or plants—are unique energy systems and will respond differently to the same treatment. Remember, too, that a client's energies will change over time, implying that what worked yesterday may not work today. Your job is to radiesthetically check and *recheck* the condition of the witness as well as the preferred treatment, then adjust your work space accordingly.

Below is a sampling of broadcasting techniques in use today. Some call for instruments; others, simply easily available diagrams. Suppliers for all such equipment, as well as addresses for more information on each technique, are listed in the resource section at the back of this book.

Magnetic Field Broadcasting

Magnetic field broadcasting is an easy and inexpensive method I first became acquainted with in the 1970s, when I began working with an instrument known as a Magnetron. This major piece of broadcasting equipment consists of a simple magnetic board inscribed with a pattern (see figure 7–1) on which the practitioner sets the broadcast. It was developed in 1977 by Dr. Christopher Hills at University of the Trees, in Santa Cruz, California.

The first step in implementing this method is to orient the Magnetron to the north so that the earth's magnetic field can booster the broadcast. Either direct sunlight or full-spectrum artificial light can also increase its effectiveness.

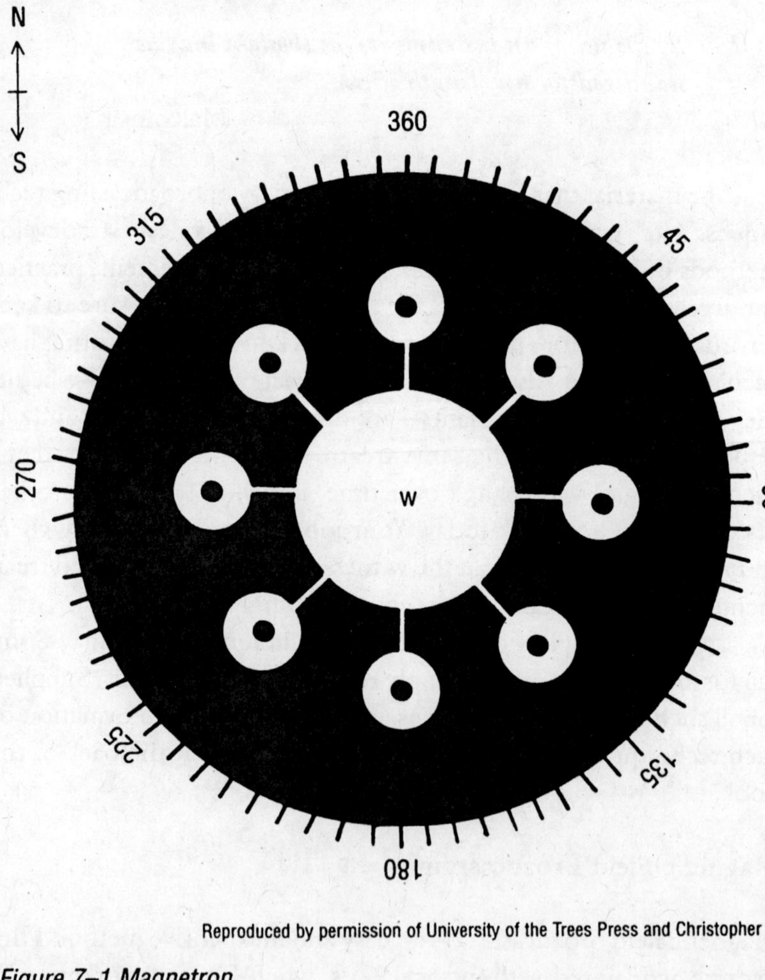

Reproduced by permission of University of the Trees Press and Christopher Hills

Figure 7–1 Magnetron

Second, using a photograph as a witness allows the broadcast materials, such as vitamins or herbs, to be placed on the site of the problem—the jaw if a tooth is the culprit, or the ankle if an injury has occurred there. If instead you decide to use hair, sputum, or some other witness, be sure to target the site of imbalance on a diagram. When using a diagram, place the witness in the central circle of the Magnetron.

Next, find the critical rotation position (CRP) of the witness by consulting your pendulum and rotating the witness until you get a strong positive swing, indicating correct orientation. The CRP was discovered by the delaWarrs, who found that each form of matter seems to have a CRP peculiar to itself—one that exists in a stable magnetic field and gives off distinctive radiations. Finding the CRP of a witness is akin to "tuning the broadcast."

The materials to be broadcast depend on what is needed and what is available. Possibilities might include Bach Flower Remedies, gems, aromas, vitamins or minerals, homeopathic remedies, or cell salts such as Nat. phos. (a regulator of the acid-alkaline balance). Upon dowsing the witness for more specific information, you may find that the client needs mint leaves for nourishing the etheric vehicle, echinacea to cleanse the blood, or cayenne to help neutralize toxins. Another possibility might be Chlorox which, because of its chemical components, helps eliminate metallic poisons. Chlorox appears to oxidize free sulfhydryl groups—potential radical formers—into disulfides that are inert to radical formation.

Another important element to consider adding to any broadcast is color. When I first started to experiment with simple broadcasting, I placed color gels over a witness, then set it in direct sunlight. Later, I replaced the gels with cathedral glass, as it seemed to conduct the energy more uniformly due, perhaps, to the gold content of the glass.

The colors themselves may be dowsed from a color list or a chart of the spectrum, looking for resonance between the witness and each color. Colors can be used either in combination or singly, and should be positioned according to your reading on the witness, the broadcast itself, and the orientation of the magnetic poles. For information on the influence of specific colors, read chapter 8.

Broadcast materials set in a clear glass container may then be placed on the witness or on whichever one of the small surrounding circles on the Magnetron pattern elicits a strong positive swing of the pendulum.

Treatment time, too, should be dowsed. Throughout, however, the broadcast must be monitored periodically and adjusted in accordance with each reading. Any time your pendulum indicates that energy is low or gone, replace the setup (see figure 7–2), focusing carefully on your procedure.

A note about the use of glass: Be sure to tap or scrape the pieces lightly together to activate the energies. The glass should then be checked for pole orientation and lined up accordingly. A strong positive swing of the pendulum each step of the way will let you know the broadcast energy is working.

In lieu of a Magnetron, you can perform magnetic field broadcasting by placing a regular magnet on top of the setup. In her book *The Science and Art of the Pendulum,* Gabriele Blackburn admits to using a sixteen-ounce horseshoe magnet with a fifty-pound pull. However large your magnet may be, make sure to orient the positive pole to the north.

Remember, there are ***no limits*** to your creativity other than those you, as an operator, impose. Use magnetic field broadcasting for the greatest good and watch wonders unfold!

Rae Methods

A wide variety of Rae cards and fine instruments are available from Magneto Geometric Applications in England. The one-well, one-card instrument called the Mark III Potency Simulator shown in figure 6–2, on page 55, is especially useful for broadcasting a gem, color, Bach remedy, or any other modality appearing on the Rae cards. With the witness in place, you could send Bach Rescue Remedy, for example, in the case of sudden trauma or suffering. These instruments can be linked up by special adapter lines to operate in tandem with each other, as well as other instruments, thereby adding to the capacity of each one. The multicard Rae instruments are equally invaluable.

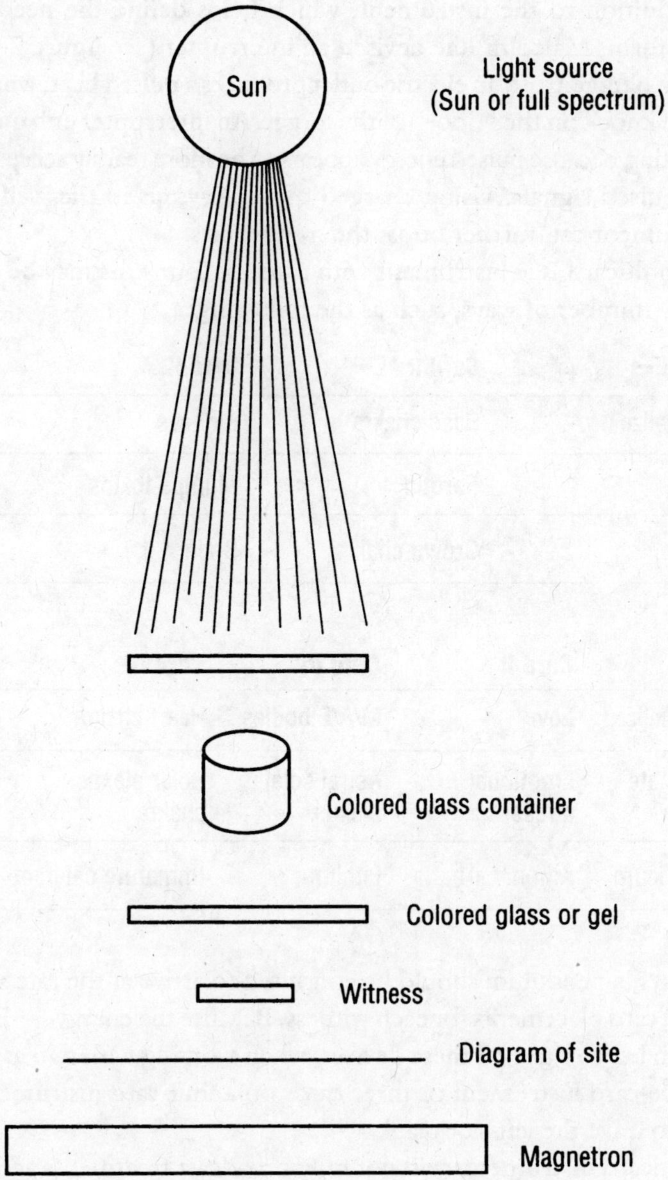

Figure 7–2 Sequence of Broadcasting Material

In addition to the instrument, which helps define the needed thought form, Malcolm Rae devised an interrupter (see figure 7–3) that when plugged into an electric outlet produces a pulsed beat, which acts like a knock on the "door" of the target. An interrupter enhances broadcasting because pulsed energy appears to be more readily accepted than unpulsed signals. Using charged quartz crystals in the well of the instrument can further boost the frequencies.

A multicard Rae instrument with three or four slots may be set up in any number of ways, such as the following:

Card I *E→	Card II *E→	Card III
1. Normalize	Base chakra	Kidneys
2. Thuja	Parotid	Mumps toxins
3. Violet	Crown chakra	Brain

Ⓦ

Card I	Card II	Card III	Card IV
1. Optimalize	Love	M/A/E bodies	Heart chakra
2. Eliminate	Emotional stress	Astral solar plexus	Solar plexus chakra
3. Causticum	Amon. carb.	Lithium	Immature cataract

Ⓦ

Always, a pendulum should be consulted to arrive at the rate settings and card placements for each witness. Because the energy—*E—runs from left to right on these devices, when working with two cards on a three-card instrument or three cards on a four-card instrument, be sure to leave the left slot blank.

Multicard instruments will not only broadcast treatments across long distances but also potentize, or increase the effectiveness of, materials for oral administration, although this function is not described in the accompanying literature. When working with Rae methods, as with others, use your creativity!

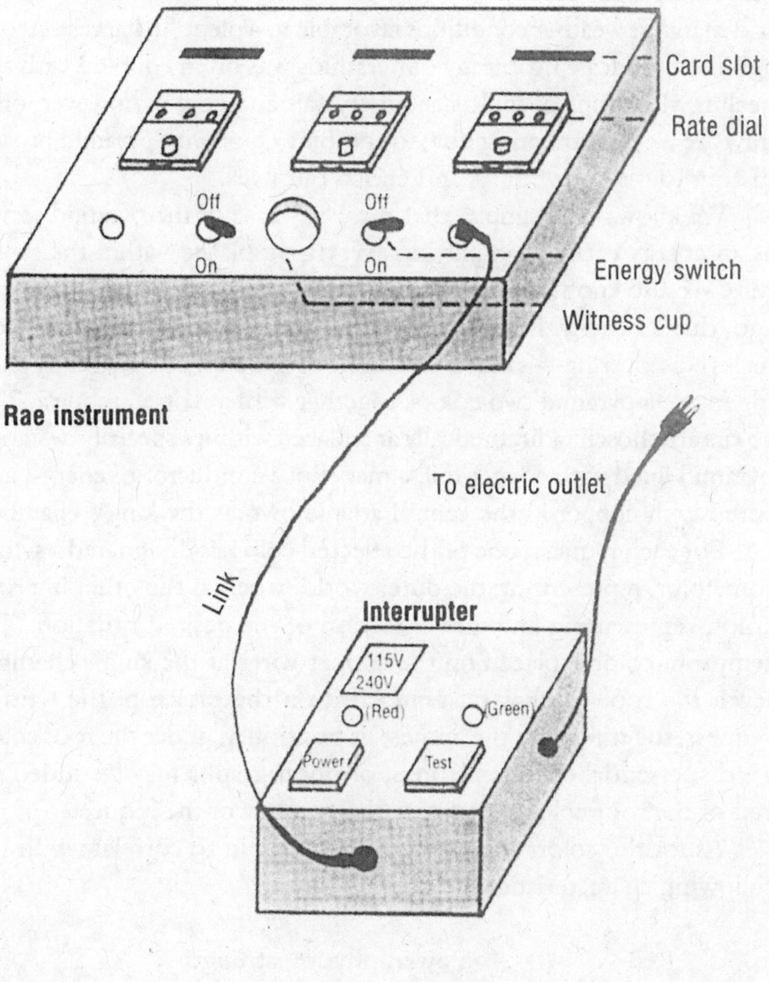

Figure 7–3 Three-Card Rae Instrument and Interrupter

Pyramids As Radionic Devices

Since ancient times, the mysterious power of pyramids has been revered and copiously studied. From documented accounts, we are aware that their energies have long been used to repair and heal the body, convert forces from the stars and planets into power for moving objects, and manifest weather conditions favorable to a plentiful harvest. Aeons ago the broadcasting energy of pyramids was often coupled with the healing vibrations of multifaceted crystals and colors; however, only now are we remembering how to combine color with pyramid broadcasting to heal our bodies and enrich our lives.

We know, for example, that the 180° base of the pyramid serves as an energy catalyst, amplifying everything placed within the structure. We also know, from the findings of Pythagoras nearly 2,500 years ago, that all energy is bipolar. What we are now discovering—or perhaps rediscovering—is that it is possible to manifest our desires by placing inside a pyramid two colors, together with a written request. The colors are chosen radiesthetically and placed within a specially designed pyramid lined with copper foil, a marvelous conductor of energy, and wired with copper in the central area known as the king's chamber.

For each request, one of thc selected colors is designated a symptom color, representing the outer world, whereas the other is a root color, representing an inner reflection of the desired situation. The symptom color is placed on the copper wires at the king's chamber level; the root color is set beneath it on the tabletop; the written request, together with the witness, is positioned under the root color. Herbs, essential oils, gemstones, or photographs may be added on top of the root color to increase the potency of the request.

As for the colors themselves, they are said to correlate with the following characteristics:

Red	Power, physical strength
Pink	Love, self-esteem
Orange	Accomplished goals
Gold	Money, security
Yellow	Communication, friendship

Yellow-green	New adventures, new beginnings
Dark green	Balance, harmony, health
Light blue	Analytical, creative
Dark blue	Wisdom in decision making
Violet	Spiritual, intuitive

Two forces give rise to a third. Hence, when the two colors are placed within a pyramid and the mind focuses clearly on the written request, miracles can happen! The results are simply signs of Pythagorean theorems in action.

Gail, a highly qualified educator, was having difficulty finding employment in a small community. Within thirty-six hours of broadcasting colors through a pyramid containing her request for a new job, she was unexpectedly approached by a nearby college faculty member and invited to submit her résumé. She was subsequently hired.

Robert frequently uses a pyramid to ask the universe for perfect tenants to occupy his rental properties. Tenants sometimes manifest within hours; if it takes days or weeks for them to appear, he claims he is satisfied knowing the universe is seeking a perfect tenant for his property.

Pets are often extremely responsive to colors broadcast through a pyramid. Jazmine, a fifteen-year-old Siamese with cataracts, appeared to heal her condition following color broadcasting.

Why does the broadcasting of colors appear to have such profound effects? Because every cell in the body resonates to the colors of the rainbow, and hence can be instantly invigorated by the external stimuli of color.

SS–Sanjeevini Healing Fragrances

Sanathana (timeless) Sai Sanjeevini (san-jee-VAN-ee) Healing Fragrances, a prayer-based healing system from India, utilizes spiritual diagrams to convert a substance into a medicine by infusing it with divine healing powers. (Although they are called "fragrances"—because they are prepared in a wooden fragranciser—Sanjeevini remedies are not aromatic.) An outgrowth of Hindu Vedantic philosophy, these solutions can be applied to people of any age and with any condition: croupy infants, injured children, and ailing elders. They are likewise effective with animals and plants. Actually, Sanjeevini-infused remedies can be broadcast as vibrations to anyone or anything in the world "and beyond." In the words of Michael Blate, executive director of the G-Jo Institute, "It is said that all dis-ease is ultimately caused by a spiritual imbalance [and] the ultimate cure of all dis-ease is to return to spiritual harmony."

This healing system is based on a simple prayer to God or the universal creative intelligence, or an affirmation. Its vibration is then transferred to a sacred diagram, or *yantra*—which is said to harness the energy—and ultimately to a medium. The diagrams can be copied for personal use; indeed, photocopies are said to be as potent as the originals. Because of the subtle energy the diagrams hold, you may want to protect them in transparent plastic sleeves when they are not in use.

The healing solution may be prepared in either a dropper glass or a plastic bottle. Begin with any medium you choose: water, medicinal alcohol, brandy, *vibhuthi* (sacred ash manifested and blessed by Sri Sathya Sai Baba in India), sugar pills, even soup. Then transfer healing vibrations from the relevant Sanjeevini diagram to the medium by placing the filled vial on the diagram, "charging" it for fifteen seconds while offering a brief prayer, *mantra* (sacred chant), or affirmation. According to Sri Sathya Sai Baba, "For those who rely on the Supreme Doctor, *his name* is the drug that cures."

> *Prayer is [a] type of mental magic which doctors of energy medicine have recommended for thousands of years.*
>
> —G-Jo Institute

The Sanjeevini solution you prepare can then be broadcast and, if desired, neutralized. To broadcast the infusion to an ailing person, animal, or plant, use the multiplication and broadcasting card shown in figure 7–4, placing the charged medium on the circle marked "sample." After writing the name of your client on a small piece of paper and placing it on the "output" circle, direct loving thoughts their way. A response may take anywhere from a few minutes to several days.

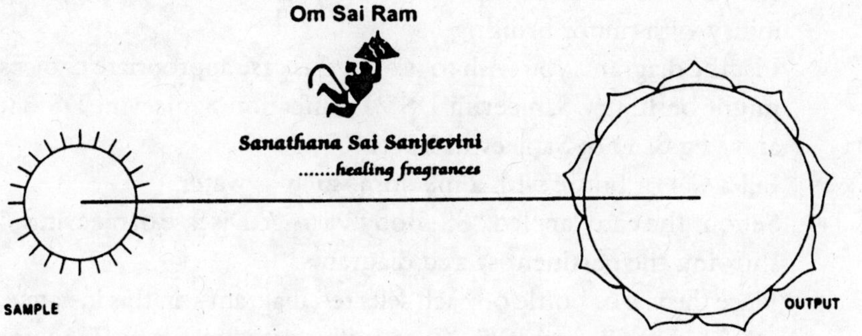

Figure 7–4 Card for Multiplication & Broadcasting of Sanjeevinis

To neutralize the healing solution, simply set it on the neutralization card shown in figure 7–5, leaving it in place for one minute. The medium is then ready for reuse.

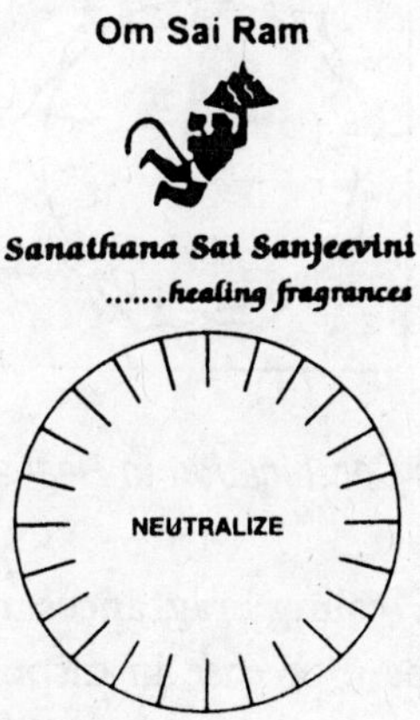

Figure 7–5 Sanjeevini Neutralization Card

According to this system, ailments call for combination remedies; hence you would dispense one of the fifty-four recommended Sanjeevini combinations. Here are instructions for preparing a combination infusion:

- Identify and list the symptoms to be treated—for example, a leg injury with minor bruising.
- List the diagrams you wish to use. In this case appropriate choices might be Injury Sanjeevini DS 71, Infection Sanjeevini DS 68, and Leg & Foot Sanjeevini BPS 27.
- Fill a vial or bottle with a medium, such as water.
- Set out the card labeled "SS–Body Parts & Disease Sanjeevinis," showing the pertinent sacred diagrams.
- Place the vial or bottle on each selected diagram—in this instance, DS 71, DS 68, and BPS 27, as is illustrated in figure 7–6—for fifteen seconds, all the while offering a prayer or affirmation. The medium is now charged with the needed healing powers and is ready for broadcasting.

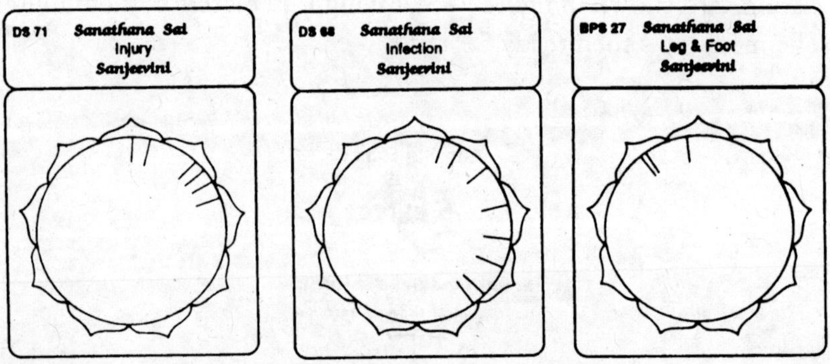

Figure 7–6 Diagrams for a Combination to Heal a Leg Injury

The SS–Sanjeevini Healing Fragrances manual lists combinations for many basic problems. For ease in dispensing them, it is a good idea to prepare these combinations in liquid or pill form, and keep them on hand as "samples." Each sample can then be used to generate new healing solutions by placing it on the "sample" circle of the multiplication & broadcasting card, setting a bottle containing fresh medium on the "output" circle, and letting them sit for thirty seconds as you offer a prayer or affirmation. The new medium will then be charged with the vibrations in the original sample.

For instance, individual samples of Shakthi (personal connectedness with God's power) Sanjeevini and Shanthi (inner peace) Sanjeevini are handy to have available, since a combination of these infusions is recommended for use in many of the healing solutions, regardless of the particular problem. Shakthi Sanjeevini (DS 113) and Shanthi (DS 114) are beneficial because improving or developing the associated spiritual and mental attributes often activates a healing (see figure 7–7).

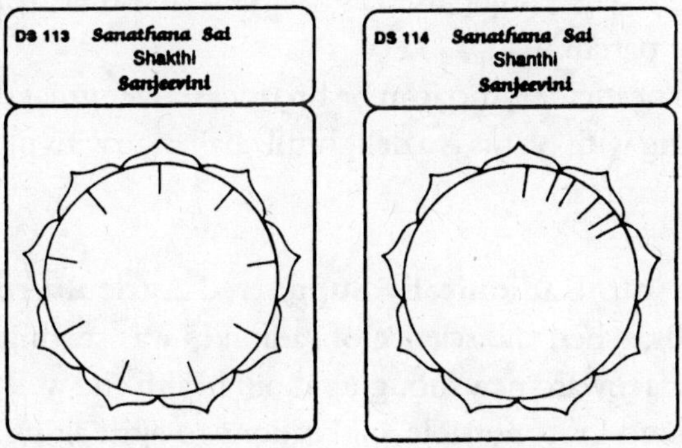

Figure 7–7 Diagrams for Shakthi Sanjeevini and Shanthi Sanjeevini

To send for the Sanjeevini cards and sacred diagrams, as well as any other equipment mentioned in this chapter, see the addresses listed in the resource section. The more you work with this broadcast system, the more convinced you will be that prayers can indeed move mountains!

Broadcasting Techniques Used in Agriculture

Plants, like humans and animals, respond well to broadcasting. Although human beings exhibit a higher level of activity, higher energy output and input, and as far as we know, a higher consciousness level, plants are composed of the same elements we are—namely, those found in the crust of the earth and in the atmosphere. Dr. C. J. Bose of India, and later Cleve Backster of the United States, proved that plants respond long distance to a variety of stimuli. Marcel Vogel, also of the United States, went so far as to demonstrate telepathic contact with his philodendron plant from a site across the Atlantic Ocean!

While working radionically with plants, I often use a leaf witness. Once, while treating an ornamental shrub that was not doing well, I placed a leaf in a two-well instrument and broadcast it back to health, resulting in greater vitality throughout the shrub. The reason for its transformation is explained by Harold Saxon Burr's finding, as described in chapter 1, that modifying any *part* of an organizational field modifies the *whole*. The sample used as a witness, in other words, was part of the larger parent field.

Natural pesticides, too, can be broadcast over great distances. All in all, working with plants is a delightful challenge with plenty of room for creative expression.

A Glimpse into Radionically Supported Agriculture

In the 1930s, when the science of radionics was stirring the cultural consciousness toward new thoughts about health and well-being, interest was sparked in its possible applications to agriculture. Soon afterward, radionic methods were tested on major agricultural problems—the pests, diseases, and weeds arising from monocrop planting.

At about the same time, agricultural technology was beginning to flood the market with pesticides, herbicides, and chemical fertilizers. Solutions were drastically needed because agriculture was becoming competitive; farmers who produced the most crops in the least amount of time were being paid the best price for them.

As it turned out, the radionically supported projects were found to have impressive results. In fact, such projects would probably be in operation today if radionic applications had been accepted by the scientific and marketing communities. But instead, radionics was classified as unexplainable, mysterious, even dangerous. The studies were suppressed, and commercial agriculture opted for dependence on the chemical management of soil and plants.

Today, radionics is once again being applied to agriculture. The past fifteen years have spawned significant interest in understanding the subtle fields and life force of soil and plants—that is, our food. One reason for this turn of events is that a concerned look at the environmental damage wrought by chemical management has prompted a number of ecological movements. Most of them have been advocating sustainable practices to soften the serious imbalances caused by chemical farming. In response, farmers are now rotating crops and integrating into their practices other cash-producing projects. As a result, organic farming is coming into its own, sparking an appreciation of the natural qualities of produce *un*treated by chemicals.

It is this setting that has built a more stable base for radionic research in agriculture. Rather than try to solve problems created by earlier farming practices, radionic practitioners are helping farmers meet the needs of soil and crops. Already, radionic tuning has proved extremely well-suited to enhancing quality, vitality, and production. Why? Because it sets the subtle field back in order, releasing stress and allowing plants to grow more quickly.

To keep the beds as resonant as possible, researchers at Little Farm Research (LFR) in Pleasant Grove, Utah, for example, apply only small amounts of natural supplements and compost. There head lettuce is typically grown in only twenty-one days. Beds of mesclun—a lettuce mix—are cut three times in the five to six weeks it takes them to grow from seeding, and one and a half pounds per square foot are cut every six to seven weeks throughout the growing season. LFR's growing season for lettuce is thirty-five to forty weeks, and when demand is high, five plantings are rotated in each sixty-square-foot bed, producing as much as 375 pounds of lettuce! This intensive growing would not be possible were it not for radionic support.

LFR, in consultation with delaWarr Laboratories, is currently developing a four-level curriculum to certify individuals in radionically supported agriculture. Researchers there see a promising future in this approach, since it produces not only fine food products but also a healthy environment for farmers. It teaches them to observe their soil and crops, understand natural laws, and adhere to their own sense of balance and order. So we see that radionic broadcasting invites a return to a simpler and more natural way of farming and gardening.

The SE-5 Biofield Spectrum Analyzer and the SE-5 Plus

One of the most exciting radionic instruments available to farmers and gardeners is the SE-5 (see figure 7–8). No larger than an average book, it runs on a 9-volt battery, or it can be adapted to household power.

This state-of-the-art instrument has remarkable capacities. Working at the subtle biofield levels, it can be used to analyze witnesses or samples, broadcast subtle energy patterns, and stimulate or potentize homeopathic remedies. In addition to functioning at all standard rates, such as those advocated by Kelly, Drown, and delaWarr, it scans for new ones at the flip of a switch; the operator simply types the desired rate or program key into the instrument's small computer. Furthermore, the SE-5 can run rates in an automatic sequential mode—a program never before available in a radionic instrument.

Operation of the SE-5 is quite simple. First, the practitioner selects a program. If gardening is chosen, seeds and soil can be analyzed, whereupon energies found lacking, such as nitrogen, can be transmitted through broadcasting.

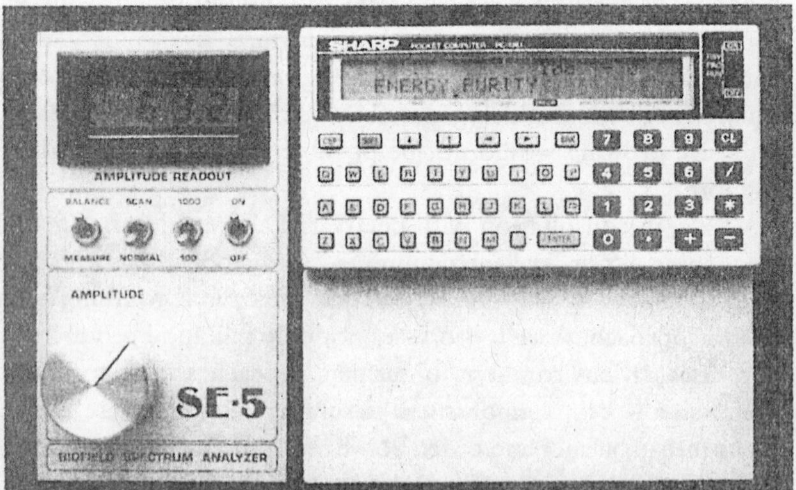

Figure 7– 8 SE–5

Vitality, states of the subtle bodies and chakras, pathogens, organ system energies, and even psychological patterns can be examined at the subtle level. Programs may be used either manually or automatically, and rates may be broadcast for a prescribed time at the discretion of the practitioner.

The SE-5 Plus, a timesaving upgrade offering a more advanced computer, is even more convenient. Like all radionic instruments, however, the SE-5 Plus focuses the mind and at some point in the practitioner's career will become unnecessary.

Into the Future with Pranamonics

> *The first question is also the final one: it is quite short, quite simple, and yet it is also the most important question which anyone could ever ask, whether of himself or of others. This question is: "What is consciousness?" Whoever traces the answer through all its levels will find himself in the end in the very presence of the universal consciousness otherwise called God.*
>
> —Paul Brunton

Pranamonics, an altogether different form of broadcasting, is a new therapy. Its name combines *prana,* breath-giving force or, in Western terms, life-force energy, with *monics,* expressing the harmonies of the cosmic dance of breath as it animates all life from the Source. Its progenitor is the extensive amount of work, inspiration, and creativity that went into the science of radionics. Like most children, however, it has taken on its own energy, purpose, and mission.

Pranamonics is classified as a spiritual healing system—with an emphasis on "spiritual." *Spirit,* as defined by esoteric wisdom, is the life breath, the cause of all manifestation; spirit lies even behind consciousness. And true health, according to Pranamonics, is a state of harmony between spirit and the matter in which it resides.

It is through the meeting of spirit and matter that we access the soul. And Pranamonics recognizes that we access the soul through the mind. Hence this healing system seeks to treat body, mind, and spirit simultaneously.

One distinguishing feature of Pranamonics is its inclusion of the mind, which is viewed as a bridge between spirit and matter. Mind's first role is to receive impressions through the five senses, and to discern and discriminate on the ground level. Mind's ultimate role—the work of the higher mind—is to respond to impressions emanating from the spiritual world. It is this aspect of the mind that is addressed in Pranamonics.

Actually, Pranamonics is designed not so much as a healing therapy, but rather as a reharmonizing of the alignment between all planes of one's existence. Upholding the essential unity of body-mind-spirit, it strives to restore the memory of Source and its perfect cosmic dance. For only in the process of reestablishing alignment between the non-manifest and the manifest does a perceptible physical healing ensue.

The development of this spiritual therapy has been laborious and at times elusive. New parameters have had to be identified, harnessed, and tested until their energetic efficacy was proved. Toward this end, three large treatment practices have been working with 200 to 400 patients apiece on trials with humans, canines, equines, and felines. Researchers are now satisfied that the extraordinary alchemy involved in aligning body, mind, and spirit does indeed have a beneficial healing effect on the physical organism.

Chapter 8

Broadcasting Healing Agents

Color Therapy, Aromatherapy, Gem Remedies, and Flower Essences

"The time has come," the walrus said,
"to talk of many things . . ."
—Lewis Carroll

In chapter 7 we explored *how* to broadcast, in all its versatility. Here we will examine *what* to broadcast. As it turns out, numerous healing agents lend themselves to radionic projection methods, only some of which are described below. In each instance, your pendulum can be used to measure settings, selections, times, and placements.

Color Therapy

The healing use of color, known as chromotherapy, began among early humans, who spent long hours outdoors in the air and sun. Their cave paintings, often rendered in vibrant hues, reflect a knowledge of the curative properties of color. As humankind became more complex, civilizations built temples—special places for healing and regenerating—where priests applied various tints and pigments as curative agents. Clearly, ancient peoples saw that just as certain herbs had specific effects on them, particular colors did, too.

The ruins of stone temples, like the caves of earlier epochs, stand as monuments to ancient human enlightenment in places such as Egypt and Greece, where color and its relation to sound and number was seen to have powerful healing influences. Some in the ancient world wrote specifically of their work in color therapy. For example, Herodotus documented his use of sunlight in the treatment of skin diseases, and Aristotle wrote a book entitled *On Color.*

Nor was the Mediterranean alone in its use of chromotherapy. Ancient red temples scattered throughout the Yucatán Peninsula, together with ochre-colored ceremonial centers decorated with splashes of blue, attest to some agreed-upon experience of color in the Americas. And in the Far East, the Chinese believed that color stimulated physical, mental, and spiritual wellness. The ancient Chinese used red material to cover what they called smallpox boxes. Evidently, the color acted as a light filter—a property revealed centuries later, in 1832, when it was found that light appeared to inhibit the progress of smallpox. In fact, it was reported that many smallpox patients wrapped in red blankets recovered without scars.

As early as the 1800s, researchers in the Western world were experimenting with the effects of color on psychological conditions. Since then, our understanding of the impact of color on all levels of healing has greatly expanded—and with it, our ability to work long-range with the various light rays.

The Mystery of Creation

In the beginning there was darkness and the Creator said, "Let there be light," and there was light . . . and then he spoke upon the waters, and the waters moved. This we learn from the biblical Book of Genesis. It describes nothing short of the essence and mystery of creation—namely, that everything visible and invisible on this planet comes out of the light. Another way of rendering this mystery is diagrammed on the following page.

Cosmic rays, gamma rays, X rays, and ultraviolet rays constitute the invisible realm of light. As light's vibration slows, we are able to perceive the rainbow of visible light we call the color spectrum. Slowing even more, the energy becomes denser as it passes through space,

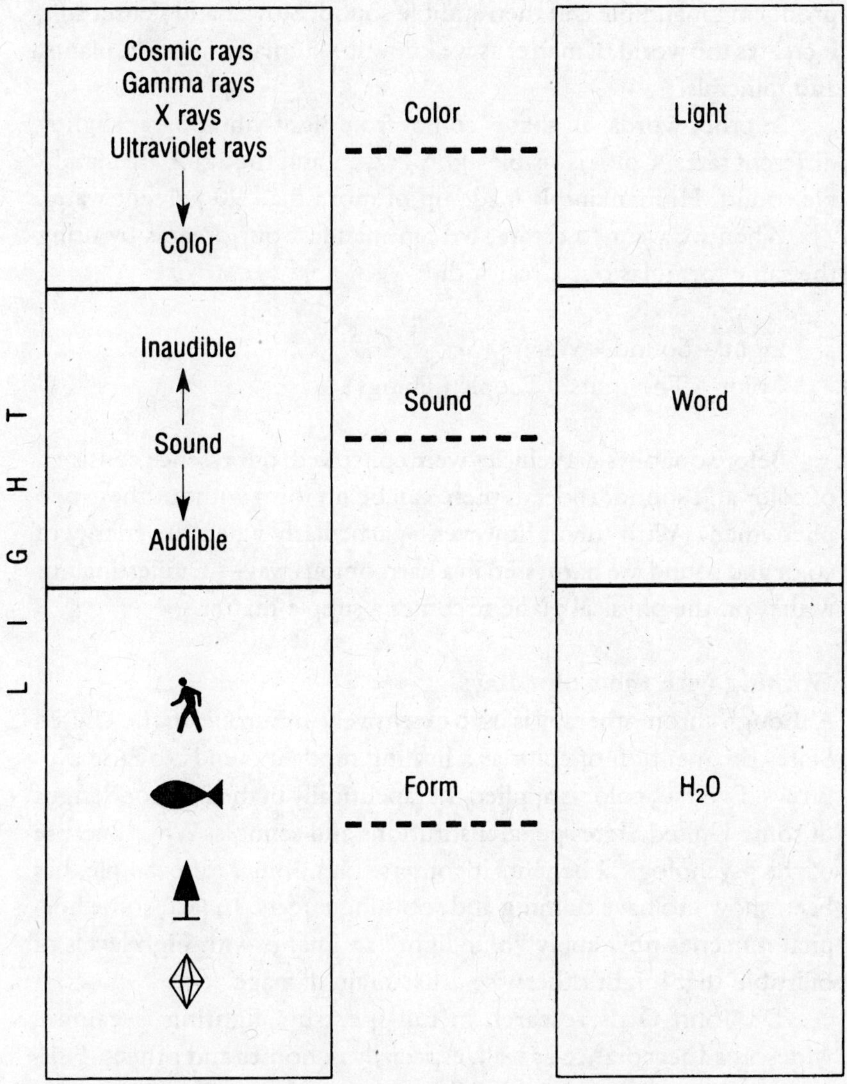

Figure 8–1 The Unfolding of Creation

producing inaudible and then audible sound. Slower and denser still, it creates the world of matter as we know it—humans, animals, plants, and minerals.

In other words, all that is comes from light vibrating at slightly different rates. Color is visible light. Prayers and thoughts are inaudible sound. Humankind is made up of more than 90 percent water.

When we want to create, we can manifest our dreams by using the same formulas our Creator did:

Light + Sound = Water
Color + Thoughts = People (Things)

Before our physical vehicles were conceived, our essence consisted of color and sound. Indeed, there can be no form without these two phenomena. With them, however—particularly when the energy of color and sound are harnessed in a harmonious way—manifesting our wishes on the physical plane becomes a simple matter.

Working with the Color Rays

Although chromotherapy is used extensively in Europe, in the United States the mention of color as a healing modality tends to raise eyebrows. Even so, color is applied therapeutically in the interior designs of some United States penal institutions and schools. Why? Because of the psychological benefits it confers. Light blue, for example, has been shown to have calming and soothing effects. In fact, some hospital nurseries now apply "blue light" to infants with high levels of bilirubin that might otherwise cause brain damage.

Dr. John Ott's research in full-spectrum lighting is gaining widespread acceptance as well, especially in homes and offices. Full-spectrum lamps are now available commercially—due, no doubt, to their remarkable impact on symptoms associated with short periods of daylight during long winters.

The Spectrum of Colors. One of the best ways to experience color is through a prism, which is what Isaac Newton did in 1666. A beam of sunlight hitting a prism is refracted into rays of colored light. These rays are seen as violet, indigo, blue, green, yellow, orange, and red—the VIBGYOR color rays mentioned in many writings— each of which is said to correspond to one of the seven major chakras. This visible spectrum produced by sunlight can be replicated by artificial light having the same light-wave content.

VIBGYOR, however, represents only an infinitesimal portion of the vibrations emanating from a light source. The other rays, although moving too quickly to be seen, still impart energy, even through a prism.

While outdoors in nature, we are exposed to the cosmic light rays as well as the visible ones that make up the color spectrum. Color itself, however, is an illusion. What we perceive as color are simply energy waves created by light shining on an object; what we see as variations in color are the degrees to which that object has absorbed the light. Several years ago a scientist friend showed me research about the colors in a hummingbird's wings. I remember well my disappointment upon learning there was no color in these feathers. It was almost like discovering there was no Santa Claus!

Interestingly, when a person is unable to see certain colors through a prism, their organism is temporarily missing these energy waves and in need of exposure to them. Healing in such instances is accomplished through chromotherapy—either by taking color in directly or by having it broadcast. The latter method is best achieved through cathedral glass, which has a gold content that seems best able to hold and conduct color energy, although other types of glass as well as color gels are also effective, as are the bright array of shades available on Rae cards. Unfortunately, traditional cathedral glass, although easy to find in Europe, is not readily available in the United States.

Chakra Chips. Recent developments in research have sparked the manufacture of three-by-three-inch Chakra Chips—pieces of cathedral glass produced in colors and shapes that correspond to the individual chakras. Lying on chips arranged on a bed or couch allows the body to absorb whatever color vibrations it needs. In the process it nourishes itself rather quickly on the physical, metabolic, emotional, mental, and spiritual levels. The chips can also be used to broadcast color, especially through the use of a radionic instrument, such as an SE-5.

One case study pertaining to the use of Chakra Chips is particularly fascinating. A clairvoyant in her late fifties had multiple health problems, including failing eyesight and hearing. After lying down and having the Chakra Chips placed on her body, she relaxed and began to experience strong sensations. At first she could feel the release of blocked energies, especially in the throat and eye areas. Then a foul odor, coming from her left ear, filled the room. The odor was eventually identified as emanations from the anesthesia she had had, beginning at age seven with a tonsillectomy and continuing with several later surgeries and the delivery of five children. When the odor was finally released, her hearing cleared.

Immediately afterward, another noxious odor filled the room, this time coming through the skin. After struggling to identify the smell, she suddenly linked it to a substance her mother had treated their hardwood floors with fifty years before. Because the substance was "poisonous," the children were not permitted to play in those rooms for twenty-four hours—which evidently was not long enough for the air to rid itself of the toxins. Following the release of *this* odor, the woman reported improved vision.

Pets, too, respond quickly to Chakra Chips. When the colors are placed next to them while resting, they are able to absorb whatever rays they need. A hyperactive animal will often calm down, and a lethargic one will become energized.

In a sense color, like a liquid, will seek its own level. It will travel wherever it is needed and then fill the void.

The Action of Colors. Chromotherapy intensifies energy at the cellular level, and it does so in two ways. It acts through the physical organism via color projections to the body, color baths, color breathing, and color drinks and food; it also acts through an awakening of consciousness. In fact, Rudolf Steiner recommended methods that act on consciousness rather than on afflictions. And indeed, color directed at the consciousness enhances physical functioning, as well as mental and emotional well-being, by bringing the entire system into balance and harmony. Cellular-level responses to color are as remarkable in the animal and plant kingdoms as they are among humans.

When broadcasting color to stimulate change in an organism, we project the vibrational rates of specific hues or combinations of them, such as green and red for immunity, or blue and violet for pain. Ending a treatment with green often harmonizes and balances the energies. Research indicates that the most potent healing colors are blue, green, and orange (combining the action of yellow and red).

According to esoteric color expert Corinne Heline, colors can be classified as soothing, stimulating, or healing, as shown in the following chart.

Action	**Physical (Emotional)**	**Mental**	**Spiritual**
Soothing	light gray-blue 2nd ray blue	olive green blue-green	azure blue to lavender-blue
Stimulating	clear red orange yellow	violet to red-violet	orchid magenta*
Healing	lavender green	rose gold-green lavender	lavender-rose magenta gold

*Magenta, the color of the transpersonal chakra, should be used with care, since this highly spiritual color is not appropriate to everyone.

Color selection will vary with the ailment. For example, one therapist I know begins sore throat treatments with blue to calm and cool; moves on to red to stimulate the healing process; and ends with blue or lavender to balance the treatment and activate the throat chakra. As always, the duration of treatment and choice of colors should be dowsed and checked regularly, since their influence can change as you proceed.

Fundamental properties of the individual colors are as follows:

Red	Stimulates circulation, heart, and hemoglobin production; boosts vitality; reduces inflammation and pain; acidifies urine
Orange	Assists lung function; ameliorates asthma and respiratory conditions; improves digestion; aids in the assimilation of calcium; enhances the action of green light waves
Yellow	Cleanses, purifies, and vitalizes; bolsters the nervous system; increases bile flow; reduces swelling; serves as an antacid (lemon shade); stimulates the bowel
Green	Heals and harmonizes; aids in liver functions; builds vitality through the eyes; stimulates the pituitary gland through the endocrines and lymphatics; serves as a germicide
Blue	Soothes inflammatory conditions and overactivity; reduces fever and tension; energizes the life force; cools; helps to antidote diarrhea; alleviates nerve ailments; serves as a depressant
Indigo	Ameliorates fever and skin problems; cools
Violet	Soothes and balances energy; dissolves discord; serves as a motor and cardiac depressant; stimulates the spleen; produces dreaminess
Blue/Violet	Alleviates pain
Green/Red	Boosts immunity
Gold	Original wave-length of light in brain; elevates mental peace and balance of the mind
Pink	Arouses compassion and love

Color	Gem	Scent	Musical Note	Possible Effects
Violet	Sapphire	Carnation Peppermint	B	Calming, purifying
Indigo	Diamond	Balsam Lavender	A	Sedating, promotes self-control
Blue	Moonstone	Lilac Sweet pea	G	Healing, soothing
Green	Emerald	Musk Narcissus	F	Balancing, relaxing, healing
Yellow	Coral	Jasmine Iris	E	Promotes mental activity, nerve balancing; laxative
Orange	Pearl	Vanilla Almond	D	Acts as a tonic, laxative
Red	Ruby	Geranium Sandalwood	C	Stimulating, vitalizing

Figure 8–2 Color-Gem-Scent-Sound Correspondences

To further enhance the action of healing colors, they can be broadcast with patterns, or with corresponding gems, scents, or musical notes. These correspondences are shown in figure 8–2.

The use of color in the treatment of human ills and discomforts is extremely simple, and its benefits far-reaching. Although either overlooked or assiduously avoided by mainstream health-care workers, in many instances it has proved to be an effective replacement for costly and often damaging drugs. Best of all, color therapy can be used by anyone, since the visible spectrum is all about us in the world of nature. Utilizing these light energies would move us a giant step ahead in achieving harmony and well-being.

Aromatherapy

Aromatherapy acts on the subtle bodies by way of scent molecules. In addition to being highly pleasing to the senses, it can have profound healing results.

Aromatherapy's essential oils, or attars, are etherically composed to produce vibrations that will activate the body's healing processes. In skilled hands these heavenly scented substances can also help correct imbalances in the mental, emotional, and spiritual bodies. As Hakim Moinuddin Chishti, ND, once said, they are "medicine for the soul."

The healing art of aromatherapy has been practiced for more than 2,000 years, beginning with such healers as Hippocrates. References to the oils are found also in the Bible, the Torah, and the Koran. Their use appears to have peaked with the mystic orders of Islam well before the end of the first century A.D. Mohammed once said that essential oils were one of his three favorite things in this world, especially musk, rose, and violet.

The word *attar*, from the Persian and Arabic, means "fragrance, odor, or essence." And what delightful fragrances some of them have! My own favorites are jasmine from Tunisia and rose.

The use of attars for physical ills was documented in the classic *Canon of Medicine* by the great Persian physician Avicenna, who also developed the steam distillation method of producing pure oils. In his work as a practitioner, Avicenna assigned values to flowers, based on their individual temperaments. These values then helped him select the most effective flower oils for treating the unbalanced temperaments of his patients.

In Europe aromatherapy began in earnest about sixty years ago, when the French cosmetics chemist René Maurice Gattefossé noticed that essential oils had an effect on the skin. He also found that many oils had antibacterial properties. More recent research in the Soviet Union has revealed that a certain eucalyptus oil can counter a type of influenza virus.

During the 1950s two well-respected European aromatherapists, Marguerite Maury and Dr. Jean Valnet, wrote books about their work.

Maury integrated oils into her holistic approach, whereas Valnet gave them orally, in the conventional medical fashion.

Today, the practice of aromatherapy continues in Europe, as it does worldwide among Muslim mystics known as Sufis. Using the attars for soul growth, Sufis associate each one with a station, or step, of the soul during its sojourn on earth—that is, they treat imbalances on the physical as well as spiritual levels with specific attars. The Sufi stations, in ascending order, are the following:

Ego
Heart
Pure spirit
Divine secrets
Proximity or nearness to God
Union with God

> *God, when he created the universe, said that the first thing he created was the Soul of Prophesy, and he said that he made it from the Absolute of His Own Light, and called it* "Nur. . . ." *It was of such luminous nature, and so burning with Light, that it began to shed drops of perspiration. And from the sweat of the Soul of Prophesy, God made the soul of the rose. This is the actual place and moment of the origin of the art and science of aromatherapy.*
>
> —Hakim Moinuddin Chishti, ND

Following is a chart of some of the most widely used oils, together with their harmonizing effects. Please understand that to truly comprehend this ancient system, intensive study with a competent teacher—only a few of which reside in the Western world—is strongly recommended.

These attars may be either applied topically in minute quantities or broadcast for the benefit of others. When storing them, be sure to protect them from light, heat, and air—preferably, in amber-colored bottles.

Amber (father of scents; affiliated with the state of proximity to God)	Ameliorates diseases associated with the heart; topically stimulates the pineal gland
Frankincense	Cleanses the aura
Jasmine	Elevates moods and lessens depression
Musk	Eases heart and sexual problems
Myrrh	Heals
Rose (mother of scents; associated with the state of union with God)	Purifies and uplifts the physical, emotional, and spiritual bodies
Sandalwood	Assists in serious meditative and spiritual practice; quiets the ego; calms sexual energies
Sweet almond	Serves as a slight stimulant and a blending oil; helps move nutrients under the skin; may protect against cancer
Violet	Provides mild healing action

Gem Remedies

For many decades Drs. Bhattacharya in Naihati, India, have been studying gems, writing about them, and broadcasting their therapeutic effects to clients around the world. Virginia Beach seer Edgar Cayce often recommended gemstones in his readings; for example, lapis lazuli was advised to impart vitality and strength. Aside from Cayce's readings, however, the healing use of gemstone vibrations has until recently been sparse in the Western world. Only now are we learning to acknowledge their curative powers.

> *Of the five kingdoms, the crystal kingdom is the most concentrated. We can become workers with the life-form if we approach them with respect. Their physical forms are only a small part of who they are, just as our form is only a small part of who we are.*
>
> —Allachaquora

Gem remedies can be taken orally or topically in tincture form, in which case they tend to be a bit more potent and fast-acting than flower essences, described on page 96. Gems can be worn as well—on clothing or, preferably, against the skin. In addition, some practitioners suggest placing a gem in pure water that the client then drinks, absorbing the vibrations of the jewel. The proper administration of gem remedies depends on individual need, so be sure to carefully check each client radiesthetically before dispensing the chosen therapy.

Gem energies can also be broadcast. In the absence of a prepared remedy, you may be able to simulate the essence of the chosen stone through the use of an instrument such as the Mark III. Rae cards are also available for a large variety of jewels.

Following is a partial list of the more familiar gems and their effects:

Amethyst	Raises personal thoughts and desires into universal realms
Aquamarine	Clears congestion from the etheric level on up
Diamond	Intensely stimulates an alignment of personal will with divine will. (Use with care.)
Emerald	Balances; attunes to the life force; clarifies decision making; increases clairvoyance and clairaudience

Gold	Stimulates expansion and warmth; serves as essence of solar energy
Moonstone	Aids understanding; serves as essence of lunar energy
Ruby	Promotes expansion; enhances vitality; aids circulation in the etheric body; promotes thermal balance
Sapphire	Stimulates transmutation of habit patterns on all levels; increases optimistic outlook
Silver	Cools; promotes reflection; serves as essence of lunar energy
Topaz	Releases etheric obstructions; aids mental focus in communications; helps alleviate spiritual depression
Turquoise	Balances emotions; relieves stress and obstructions to rhythmic flow

Figure 8–3 shows major gems on a radiesthesia chart, which can be dowsed any time you wish. As always, begin by placing the witness where indicated.

Flower Essence Remedies

These products, which include the well-respected Bach Flower Remedies, are now familiar to most health-care practitioners. They are highly effective and can be broadcast, taken orally, or applied topically. They can also be used to treat animals and plants.

The original Bach Flower Remedies were developed in the 1930s by Dr. Edward Bach, a British physician. His medical work had not satisfied him until he pursued homeopathy, a discipline that regards the patient as the most important factor in determining a cure.

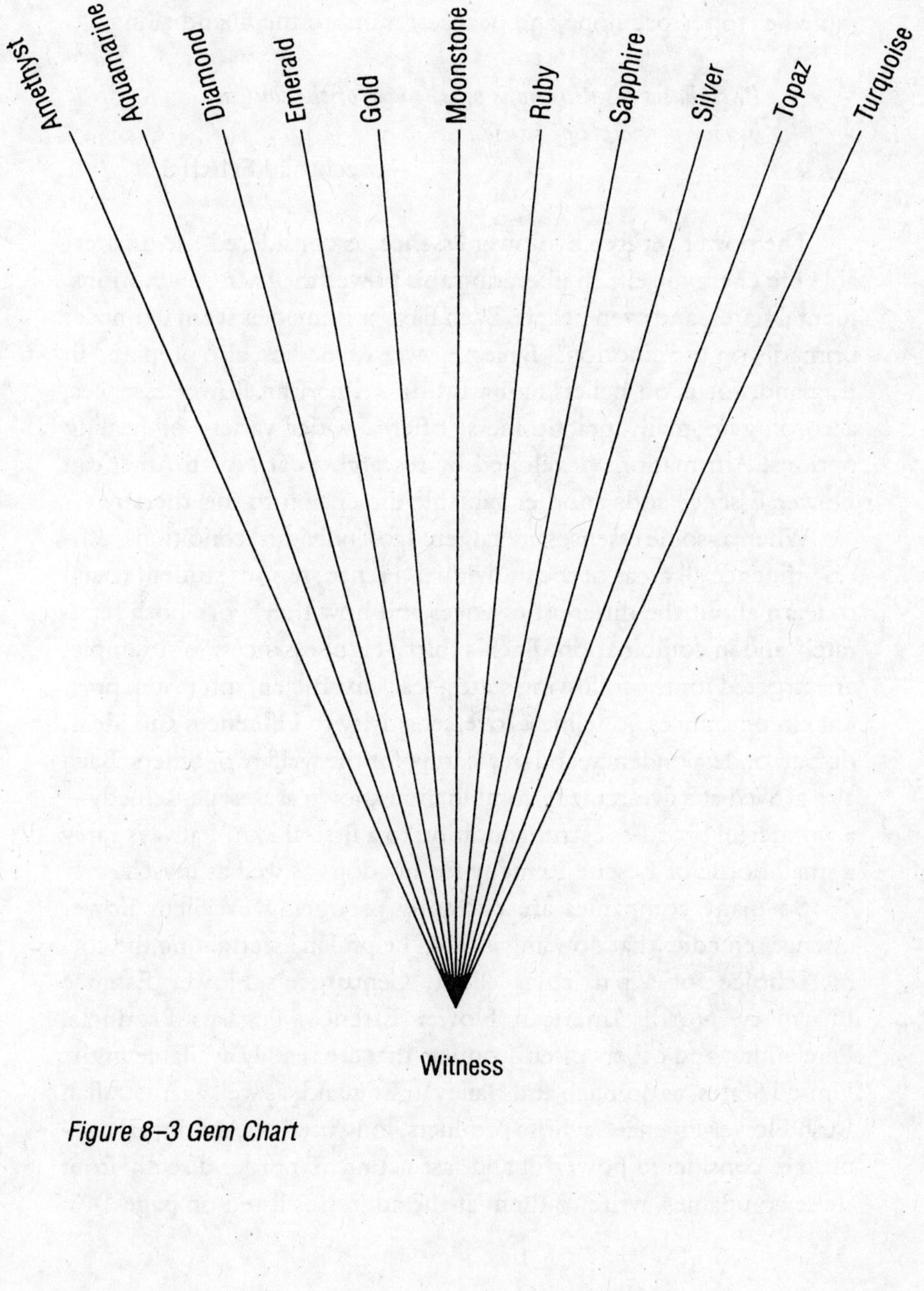

Figure 8–3 Gem Chart

Eventually, Dr. Bach turned to nature and the plant kingdom for quick remedies to restore hope and peace of mind to the ill and ailing.

> *Bach bases his diagnosis on the law of the soul, a higher principle of cause . . .*
>
> —Mechthild Scheffer

The power set free by flower essences is considered the unalterable life energy itself. In liberating this power they act on emotions, mental states, and even beliefs. Bach Flower Remedies seem to impact primarily on the emotions; Bailey Flower Remedies, also prepared in England, focus on beliefs and attitudes. American flower essences, according to many practitioners, offer a wider variety of healing options. Affirmations developed by researchers at North American Flower Essence adds another valuable dimension to this therapy.

Whereas some essences are targeted for individual conditions, others influence all areas of the individual. Hence, serious students need to learn about the different essences and how they work both separately and in combination. Bach's thirty-eight essences, for example, are targeted for the following states: fear, insufficient interest in present circumstances, loneliness, oversensitivity to influences and ideas, despair or despondency, and overcaring for the welfare of others. Bach also arrived at a five-remedy combination known as Rescue Remedy—a wonderful broad-spectrum addition to a first-aid kit. I always carry a small bottle of Rescue Remedy for my dogs as well as myself.

So many companies are currently producing excellent flower essence remedies that dowsing is often helpful in ascertaining the correct choice for a particular client. Centurgee's Flower Essence Pharmacy, North American Flower Essence, Pegasus Products, Perelandra, and others offer products that are readily available in the United States, as do Bach and Bailey in England, as well as Australian Bush Flower Essences, whose products, long used by Aboriginal people, are considered powerful and fast-acting. To order directly from these companies, write to them at the addresses listed on page 143.

> *Well may* Isis Unveiled *tell us that sounds and colors are all spiritual numerals; nor is that all, for odors, metals and planets are equally spiritual numerals. Each planet (or spiritual plane) has relation to a metal or color. These again are in correlation with a corresponding odor and sound. The sphere of the aura that surrounds every human being has one very important fold, or layer, which invariably bears the color of the metal and planet to which that individual has most affinity; and it is on this layer that the magnetic part of odors and all sound vibration impinges.*
>
> —*The Theosophist*, vol. 7

Chapter 9

Energy Medicine

Homeopathy and Schüssler Cell Salts

The electromagnetic field of the human body can be considered its "dynamic plane"—a plane of inconceivable complexity which nevertheless conforms to laws and principles grounded in electromagnetic concepts of resonance, harmony, reinforcements, and interference. These laws and principles, therefore, are the basis of the new energy medicine.

—George Vithoulkas, MIH

Energy medicine influences an organism's chemistry and structure by interacting with it on more subtle levels. It heals by stimulating and strengthening the body's own vital force mechanism through materials selected for their energy-imparting properties. Its aim is to change the body's environment by paying close attention to what the organism is doing and trying to assist in the endeavor. A well-chosen homeopathic remedy or Schüssler cell salt, sometimes called tissue salt, can effectively accomplish this goal by balancing the body's electromagnetic fields, thereby eliminating the cause of disorder. Because of the energy characteristics of homeopathic and cell salt materials, the radionic practitioner will find in each of them a near-perfect partner.

Homeopathic Remedies

> *When Dr. Hahnemann first formulated the concept of homeopathy, he gave to the world an extremely effective system of therapy, which has survived the test of time incredibly well.*
>
> —Malcolm Rae

Homeopathic remedies usually come from animal, vegetable, or mineral sources. They are given in minute doses—dilutions prepared through a traditional, proven process of potentization, or dynamization. Homeopathic potencies, the latent energy in the remedies, are generally expressed in terms of the decimal scale (designated by the letter *x*) or the centesimal scale (indicated by a *C*). Dosage rules are governed by the Law of Similars, which states that the greater the resemblance between one's symptoms and a remedy's proven pattern, the stronger the needed dose or dilution.

Millesimal potencies of 1M or higher, because of their possibly far-reaching effects, should be prescribed only by a homeopathic physician. Lower potencies in the 6x–30x range, however, may be safely administered by less experienced practitioners. A chart for dowsing potencies is pictured in figure 9–1.

To be effective, a homeopathic remedy must harmonize with the client's susceptibility level. It can then help bring about a cure by stimulating the organism's vital force and defenses. Administered correctly, such a remedy will produce no side effects. Because of the potent energetic materials contained in homeopathic medicines, however, they should be disseminated with *knowledge of* and *respect for* the recommended indications and doses.

Homeopaths look for the *total* picture of symptoms and signs—physical, mental, and emotional—only some of which represent the body's overt attempts to heal itself. After careful consideration, a practitioner will select a remedy that in its crude state produces similar symptoms and signs. The energy of the chosen remedy, if it is to stimulate the organism's self-healing potential, must resonate energetically with the client. A good way to check for resonance is to

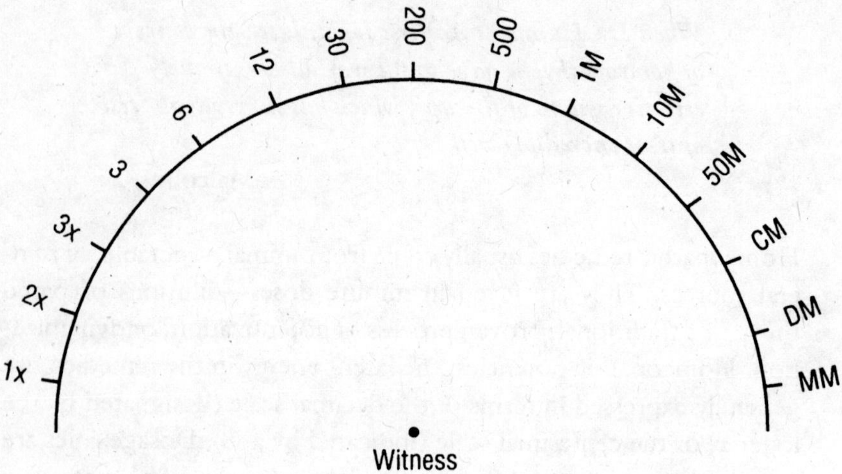

Figure 9–1 Homeopathic Potency Chart

dowse for the presence of a harmonic ray between the client witness and the remedy.

The word *homeopathy,* coined in 1826, comes from *homeo,* meaning "similar" and *pathos,* meaning "suffering." Its basic tenet—"Like cures like"—implies that homeopaths prescribe remedies that produce the same effect as the conditions themselves, thereby cooperating with the body's defenses. Success is often immediate and dramatic.

> *Since allopathic drugs are never selected according to the Law of Similars, they inevitably superimpose upon the organism a new drug-disease which then must be counteracted by the organism.*
>
> —Samuel Hahnemann, MD

Practitioners of radionics and radiesthesia, already familiar with the impact of vibrational rates on various dis-ease imbalances, neatly fit the homeopathic mode. In fact, Malcolm Rae's Mark III potency preparer shown in figure 6–2 on page 55, well-proven internationally, is able to simulate homeopathic remedies, and is packaged together with more than 2,000 remedy cards. A two-well model of this instrument, also widely available, will produce a "clone," or duplicate of an already prepared remedy, although remedy preparation itself usually takes only six to ten minutes. Best of all, these small portable instruments are remarkably effective at broadcasting homeopathic remedies to bring about healing at a distance.

One of the many unique features of homeopathy is its capacity to antidote the devastating effects of some allopathic drugs, particularly those present in vaccinations. The practice of vaccinating, although often associated with the Law of Similars, is not aligned with homeopathy's insistence on the careful selection of remedies based on an individual's symptoms and signs. On the contrary, vaccination is the administration of a foreign substance to *everyone,* regardless of their state of health or individual sensitivities. This indiscriminate practice has led to a condition known as "vaccinosis" and found to underlie certain chronic disorders to such an extent that it has been incorporated into some radionic analysis forms.

Vaccinations change the organism's electromagnetic vibrations and balance, as do any invading microorganisms. Depending on the individual's constitution, symptoms may or may not arise years later; and if they do, they may not necessarily be identified as vaccine related. Problems may also arise rapidly, as in childhood reactions to the pertussis vaccine and the widespread outbreak of Guillan-Barré syndrome, a neurological disorder that erupted on the heels of the federal swine flu vaccination campaign in the mid-1970s.

Vaccinosis has appeared after smallpox, rabies, measles, polio, flu, typhoid, paratyphoid, and tetanus shots. Tetanus vaccines have also been suspect in adult nerve-muscular disorders.

In preparing to administer a homeopathic treatment for vaccinosis, the practitioner would look for a remedy with a similar rate so as to neutralize the offending microorganism or disease toxin. The remedy *Variolinum,* for example, will often neutralize smallpox vaccinosis. Moreover, giving a remedy for tetanus or tuberculosis vaccinosis, which have the same rate, may be tantamount to committing a "double murder."

Homeopathy is a highly effective therapy primarily because it supports the body's own vital force. Indeed, the British royal family has for decades entrusted its health care to this energy medicine. In fact, it is said that Queen Elizabeth II travels with a well-worn box containing a large supply of homeopathic remedies for herself and her family.

To be a really good classical homeopath requires years of study and practice. A medical background, however, is not necessary and may even prove to be an impediment. In many countries lay homeopaths are allowed to practice on a par with medical professionals.

> *The overall health of the human population is deteriorating either because of the employment of allopathic therapeutics or in spite of it . . . . It remains my contention that our health is being compromised by the widespread allopathic drugging in effect.*
>
> —George Vithoulkas, MIH

The following homeopathic remedies are generally recommended for inclusion in a home remedy kit, which can be purchased already assembled from a homeopathic supplier. Note that each of these remedies has many applications in addition to those listed here. If you are interested in working homeopathically, by all means invest in a selection of remedies, a homeopathic *Materia Medica,* and J. T. Kent's *Repertory,* together with other selected references. Also consider enrolling in a study course. For a listing of homeopathic sources of information as well as suppliers, see the resource section at the back of this book.

Aconitum napellus (Monkshood)	For trauma with *fear,* restlessness, panic, or a combination of all three; pain and shock from foreign objects in the eye; high temperature, dry skin, and intense thirst associated with colds of *sudden onset.*

Apis mellifica (Honeybee)	For stings, sunburn, or hives; itchy, irritated skin that is bright pink with swelling and burning.
Arnica montana (Leopard's bane, mountain daisy)	For pain associated with mental or physical trauma; sprains; painful healing breaks; bruising; muscular aches; the effects of shock. *A versatile healing agent.*
Arsenicum album (White oxide of arsenic)	For gastrointestinal upsets, vomiting, or diarrhea from food poisoning; skin rash of ***sudden onset*** improved by heat.
Belladonna (Deadly nightshade)	For colds of ***sudden onset*** with sore throat, high temperature, facial sweating, congestion, and throbbing blood vessels.
Bryonia (Wild hops)	For discomfort from overeating; injury with intense pain upon movement.
Calendula officinalis (Marigold)	For cuts, abrasions, minor bleeding, or sunburn. Also available in ointment, tincture, and lotion form. *A great healing agent.*
Carbo vegetabilis (Vegetable charcoal)	For digestive problems; distension of the upper abdomen; flatulence after wine and fatty foods.
Chamomilla (German chamomile)	For relief of pain and irritability in children who are teething.
Cocculus indicus (Indian cockle)	For travel sickness with nausea and dizziness; insomnia due to stress.
Coffee cruda (Unroasted coffee)	For insomnia and restlessness due to exhaustion or excitability; decelerated nervous and vascular activity.

Hypericum (St. John's wort)	For trauma involving nerve pain due to tooth extraction, a crushed finger, or needle pricks; pain aggravated by touch or movement.
Ipecacuanha (Ipecac root)	For persistent nausea and vomiting; diarrhea; hypersalivation with a clean uncoated tongue.
Ledum (Marsh tea)	For accidents involving punctures, black eyes, cuts, or stings; alleviates shooting pains, particularly when wounded parts are cold.
Nux vomica (Poison nut)	For conditions brought on by modern living, such as discomfort from excessive drinking and eating. *The greatest of polycrests* (in which most symptoms are similar to those of common diseases).
Rhus toxicodendron (Poison ivy)	For ruptured ligaments and tendons around joints, especially when better with motion.
Ruta graveolens (Rue bitterwort)	For trauma to torn and wrenched tendons, bruised bones, or tennis elbow, particularly when improved by motion; eyestrain.
Sepia (Inky juice of cuttlefish)	For menstrual and menopausal problems, including hot flashes.
Sulphur (Sublimated sulphur)	For preventing a full-blown flu; decreasing the duration and severity of flu symptoms.
Symphytum officinal (Comfrey knitbone)	For trauma to the eye or cheek, reducing fracture pain, or healing a bone following a blow to the face.

Thuja occidentalis (Arbor vitae)	For common warts; frequent, sudden urination; some ill effects of vaccination, particularly in dogs.
Veratrum album (White hellebore)	For voluminous amounts of diarrhea with cramps, cold sweating, and malaise; vomiting with violent retching.

The Twelve Schüssler Biochemic Cell Salts

The Schüssler cell salts, or tissue salts, are another energy medicine exceedingly helpful to the practitioner of radionics and radiesthesia. Like homeopathic remedies, they are given in tiny doses prepared in much the same way. Wilhelm H. Schüssler, the German doctor who formulated these remedies in 1873, insisted that they not be confused with homeopathic nosodes, but rather regarded as a therapeutic system of their own.

Interestingly, the twelve salts are constituents of many well-known remedies derived from the vegetable kingdom. Each one also works well with certain homeopathic remedies. One of their distinguishing features is that they are said to be aligned with signs of the zodiac.

These inorganic mineral salts are extremely important, if not essential, to a balanced human body. Why? Because each cell in the body contains the twelve salts which, in proper quantities and proportions, affect the structure and vitality of the organs. Dr. Schüssler believed that any depletion in mineral salts contributing to a disturbance in the molecular action of a cell constitutes disease. This disease state, he said, could be remedied through the introduction of minute amounts of the salts.

All twelve salts are safe, nontoxic, and non–habit forming when used according to the directions. They can be given separately or, for some conditions, in premixed combinations—both of which are available in most natural food stores and homeopathic supply houses. The Schüssler cell salts are often effective in first aid as well, and in healing at a distance.

Below is a brief description of the cell salts, their major actions, and their associations with the zodiac. Following this list is a cell salt selection chart for dowsing purposes (figure 9–2).

Astrological Sign	Biochemic Salt	Action
Cancer	Calc. fluor. (Calcium fluoride)	Gives elasticity to tissues; aids circulation.
Capricorn	Calc. phos. (Calcium phosphate)	Promotes the formation of sound bones and teeth; relieves teething pain; heals bone; aids in food assimilation.
Scorpio	Calc. sulph. (Calcium sulphate)	Purifies the blood; ameliorates skin eruptions.
Pisces	Ferr. phos. (Iron phosphate)	Aids in oxygen distribution. A constituent of red blood cells.
Gemini	Kali. mur. (Potassium chloride)	Controls plaque in blood vessels; helps form fibrin from albumin; remediates colds and coughs.
Aries	Kali. phos. (Potassium phosphate)	Nourishes the nerves; alleviates headaches.
Virgo	Kali. sulph. (Potassium sulphate)	Aids in healthy formation of epidermal tissue; relieves bronchial coughs.

Leo	Mag. phos. (Magnesium phosphate)	Acts on nerve and muscle fibers; soothes cramps and neuralgia.
Aquarius	Nat. mur. (Sodium chloride)	Controls distribution of water in the tissues.
Libra	Nat. phos. (Sodium phosphate)	Regulates the acid-alkaline balance; neutralizes hyperacidity.
Taurus	Nat. sulph. (Sodium sulphate)	Eliminates excess water; stimulates liver and pancreas.
Sagittarius	Silica-Silicea tera (Silica oxide)	Aids in elimination of wastes; combats inflammation, boils, and brittle nails.

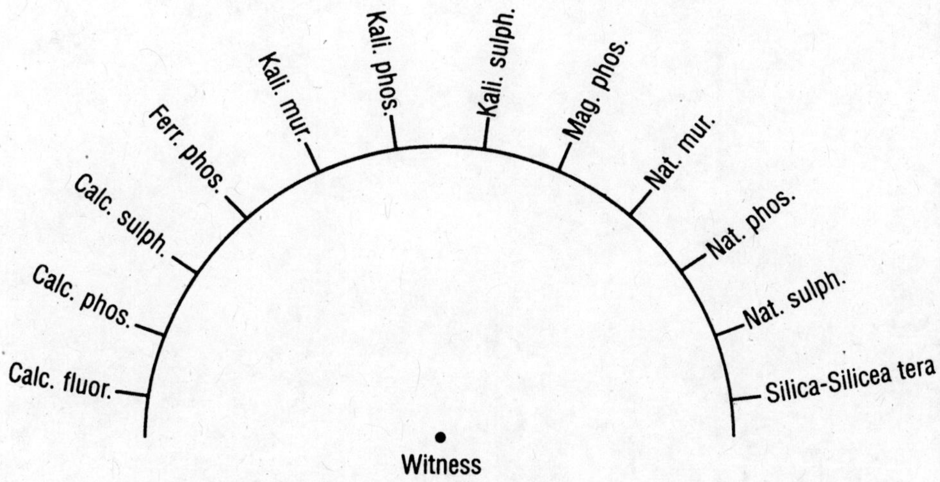

Figure 9–2 Cell Salt Selection Chart

Homeopathy and Schüssler cell salts are only two forms of energy medicine. No doubt, many more self-healing energy modalities will be readily available in the future, inviting individuals to take back the responsibility for their health and well-being. This reclamation alone can return energies to an organism attempting to restore balance. After all, it is mind, rather than matter, that is the essential reality, for mind gives rise to matter.

> *It is man's mind that is really responsible for his illness or health. He himself is the cause or motivator of either. So when it comes to healing or curing, the necessary faith has to be created within his mind for the purpose.*
>
> —Sri Sathya Sai Baba

Chapter 10

The Seven Cosmic Rays

Unlocking the Soul's Purpose

Man, know thyself.
—Plutarch

The seven rays are among the most intriguing forces of energy. They were introduced to radionic practitioners more than twenty years ago by David V. Tansley, DC, as a means for analyzing human beings, thereby opening many doors to the healing community. Through the seven ray system we are now able to better understand the progression of individuals at this "earth school" in which we are all enrolled.

In my own work with the seven rays, I have repeatedly found clients at last able to bypass blocks that have existed for years. Health-care practitioners of all sorts, especially psychologists and psychiatrists, would do well to include this technique in their work, for in the hands of a skilled advisor the rays can be true cosmic enlighteners.

The seven rays of energy may be viewed as building forces for everything in the manifested universe. Their essential nature, together with their effects on human beings, although currently under study, contains elements that human consciousness cannot comprehend.

Each ray has unique characteristics, and like everything else, each characteristic has its positive and negative aspects. The negative ones—termed weaknesses, vices, and glamours—are distractions or obstacles that must be dealt with, worked through, or overcome if progress is to be made.

Each human being, as we saw in chapter 1, is a microcosm of the universal plan. The rays, sythesizers of all universal energies, supervise the implementation of this blueprint. As if responding to a musical chord from the spheres that triggers a chain reaction in things complementary to it, the rays initiate the building of the universe from greater to lesser images.

Esoteric knowledge passed on to us through the centuries seems to agree with this assessment. Furthermore, it is said that all the information pertaining to the universal blueprint has been written and handed down, and is available to those whose consciousness is able to decipher it. In addition, present-day physicists maintain, based at least partially on the body of existing data, that unidentifiable and unmeasurable forces do exist. Such forces would no doubt include the seven rays, as well as other enigmatic aspects of radionics and radiesthesia.

Vibrational Activity of the Rays

The seven rays are in constant motion, cycling about in dynamic gyrations as they proceed on their individual courses. We may envision them as participants in a great cosmic dance, ever flowing and moving, as ancient Hindus once said of such "dancers"; others have called this activity the yin and yang of existence. At certain times and in certain regions of the planet, some rays appear more dominant than others, bringing their intensity and characteristics to the forefront of human consciousness.

It has also been said that each human energy system tends to be a composite of the labor of several rays. This situation can at times lead to problems, since an individual's personality may vibrate in unison with one ray and their physical body with another. Or the mental, astral, and emotional bodies of the personality may carry the vibrations of different rays, thereby blocking expression of the soul's purpose.

One way to help such an individual discover the evolutionary path they are to travel is by conducting a thorough analysis of the rays that play a part in their makeup. I have sometimes found it helpful to have a client go through the various ray characteristics described later in this chapter to identify the building forces that pertain to them. To assist in this preliminary analysis, we use the simple work sheet shown in figure 10–1. Try it for yourself if you like.

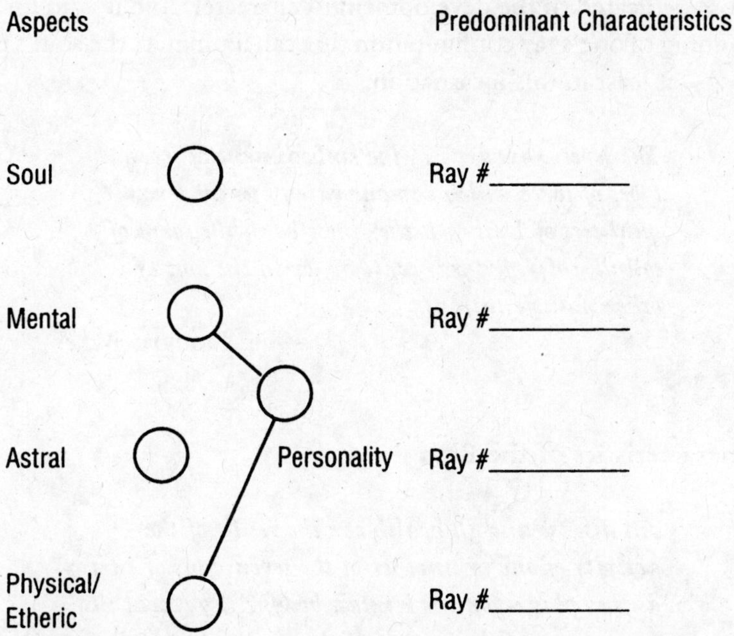

Directions: Study each of the seven cosmic rays, then list the characteristics that seem to pertain to the aspects of your being in your present state of evolution. When you feel you have found a match for one aspect, write the ray number in the appropriate circle. After filling in all five circles, dowse your rays to see how closely the information matches the answers you have arrived at. Compare the differences and reflect on them. Refer often to this work sheet to familiarize yourself with the rays and how they influence your development.

Figure 10–1 Cosmic Ray Self-Evaluation Work Sheet

The seven rays are divided into two groups: rays of aspect and rays of attribute. The *rays of aspect* (numbers one, two, and three) are major rays of will and purpose; the rays of *attribute* (numbers four, five, six, and seven) are minor rays of quality and character. The minor rays are combinations of the major ones, and hence overlapping qualities are often observed. Despite the overlaps between characteristics influencing the subtle and material levels of existence, however, lives devoted to the unfolding of the soul's purpose differ markedly from those dedicated to the development of character. And it is an understanding of one's ray configuration that can illuminate the soul's purpose—at least in this incarnation.

> *The seven rays are . . . the embodiment of seven types of force which demonstrate to us the seven qualities of Deity whether these be in the form of sound, color, fragrance, taste, or in the host of other manifestations.*
>
> —Dr. Douglas Baker

Characteristics of the Rays

> *All disease and ill health are the result of the activity of one or another of the seven types of energy as they play upon the human body. All physical ills emerge out of the impact of these imperfect energies as they make their impact, enter into, pass through the centers in the body. In addition, most human disorders seem to begin on the emotional or astral level. There the ray relation to chakras differs slightly from that on the etheric level.*
>
> —Alice A. Bailey

The individual ray characteristics are profiled in the next portion of this chapter. Characteristics that are listed were compiled from several sources, including the works of Alice Bailey, the teachings of David

Tansley, and Geoffrey Hodson's *The 7 Human Temperaments.* These profiles, you will note, contain conflicting material on color correspondences and musical notes. As always when interpreting esoteric findings, follow your own guidance about which approach seems best.

According to both Pythagoras and Isaac Newton, each note of the descending C-major scale corresponds energetically to a specific color, as follows:

B—Violet
A—Indigo
G—Blue
F—Green
E—Yellow
D—Orange
C—Red

Alice Bailey, in *Esoteric Psychology I,* lists both esoteric and exoteric colors for each ray.

In my own work with ray analysis I have found that meditating on the soul-ray symbol, musical note, and ray color tend to "bring in" the predominating soul-ray influence, overcoming blocks to its expression. We are here, after all, to fulfill our soul's purpose, and what better way is there to elicit this information than by sounding its vibratory note?

Radiesthesia, too, can help us determine resonant techniques and ray configurations. The pendulum operator must be very clear, however, when attempting such determinations.

Use of the rays in radionic analysis, as is demonstrated in Tansley's work, allows the practitioner to gain valuable insights into a client. Even so, the seven rays should be studied carefully to avoid drawing conclusions that may be invalid and possibly damaging. Tansley's books are highly recommended for delving more deeply into the esoteric aspects of the seven ray system of analysis.

As you study the following profiles, you will find that certain rays have an affinity for another ray—such as one and seven, two and six, and three and five. Hodson has proposed that the first three rays are the "spiritual ensoulment" of the last three, all of which impact on form, and that the fourth ray acts as a bridge between both "the related pairs and the two sets of three."

The rays also govern specific chakras. In fact, they are the *energies* that flow through these centers of force, and they are the programmers as well. In the process of penetrating all the subtle bodies, however, the rays' functions change. Tansley, after gleaning insights from Bailey's *Chakras, Rays and Radionics,* noted shifts in rays three, four, and seven as they pass from the etheric body to the finer astral body, as is indicated below. Since the astral body is where most human troubles begin, treating at this level is often enormously helpful.

Ray	**Etheric Aspect of Chakra**	**Astral Aspect of Chakra**
1	crown	crown
2	heart	heart
3	throat	sacral
4	brow	base
5	sacral	throat
6	solar plexus	solar plexus
7	base	brow

In recent years new rays have come to the attention of numerous channels in the United States and abroad. This information is best approached with caution, as it, unlike the esoteric literature of the seven rays, has not yet been subjected to decades of scrutiny. At the same time, do keep in mind the possibility that information is now "coming through" to help accelerate human evolution and that some of this influx may well include additional cosmic forces to work with. Essentially, the new information points to the existence of five or more rays that appear to serve not as building forces but rather as cleansing light forces to assist us in establishing contact with the higher realms during the new millennium.

> *When the hypothesis of the soul is accepted, when the nature of the spiritual energy which flows through the soul is admitted, and when the mechanism of the force centers is studied, we shall make rapid progress towards knowledge.*
>
> —Alice A. Bailey

Profiles of the Seven Rays

The influence of each of the rays is summarized on the following pages. After studying their characteristics, identify the ray that plays a prominent role in your life—and don't be surprised if you find more than one. Invite your clients to read through the profiles and select those that feel most familiar to them. To check for accuracy, dowse all hunches. And remember that a person's predominating soul-ray may change over time. This exercise alone is sure to deepen your understanding of your clients and their understanding of themselves.

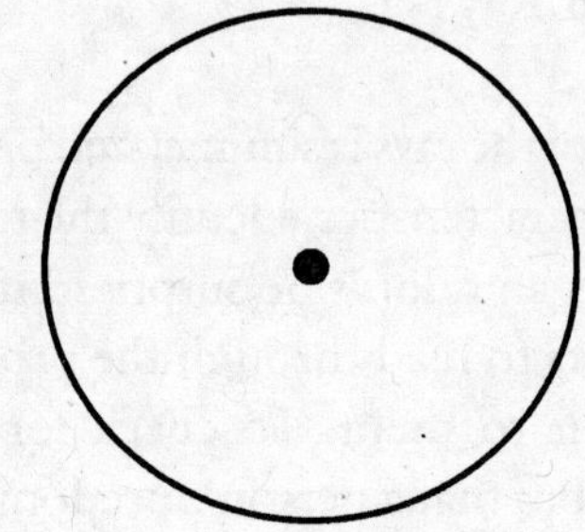

First Ray

It is the will *which initiates.*
—Alice A. Bailey

Qualities:	Power, will, courage, self-reliance
Type:	Ruler, soldier, explorer, statesman, leader
Greatest good/evil:	Power, strength/Weakness, surrender
Driving impulse:	To conquer, attain, find ultimate reality; often at best in adversity
Highest attainment:	Victory; omnipotence, exhilaration over power, kingship, dominion over nature and outer self; will as a selfless, effortless expression
Teaching method:	Drive home the truth; leave pupil to stand alone; exile
Means of achievement:	Concentration of will forces; overpowering; destroying; pronouncement of

	own will as the highest authority, of own way as The Way; discipline of subordinates
Weaknesses, vices, or glamours:	Tyranny, self-pride, domination, contempt, selfishness, thirst for power, rigidity, extravagance, individualism
Sources of suffering:	Defeat, degradation, displacement, humiliation, subordination, exile
Related religion:	Hinduism
Art:	Dancing; the creator of dances
Gem:	Diamond
Colors:	White-fire, electric blue, vermilion, orange
Musical note:	"Do"

Second Ray

It is the Christ or Vishnu aspect; it is the sentient consciousness aspect of deity in form.
—Alice A. Bailey

Qualities:	Universal love and wisdom, insight, intuition, philanthropy, sense of oneness, spiritual sympathy, cooperation
Type:	Sage, healer, teacher, reformer, lover of fellow humans and all life
Greatest good/evil:	Wisdom and love/Hate
Driving impulse:	To save, illumine, teach, share, heal
Highest attainment:	Full and unbroken realization of unity; imparting of wisdom; omniscience; continual expansion of the experience of unity
Teaching method:	Share knowledge, illumine from within, bestow happiness

Means of achievement:	Intuitive insight and perception, self-illumination, winning over, negotiating, nonresistance, turning the other cheek
Weaknesses, vices, or glamours:	Sentimentality, sensuality, impracticality; unwise self-sacrifice for others (undermining their self-reliance and increasing their selfishness); accentuating life to the neglect of form
Sources of suffering:	Heartbreak, loneliness, isolation, exclusion; neglect, broken faith and trust; coldness, disloyalty, misjudgment
Related religion:	Buddhism
Art:	Music, the harmonizing preserving art
Gem:	Sapphire
Colors:	Azure blue, indigo
Musical note:	"Sol"

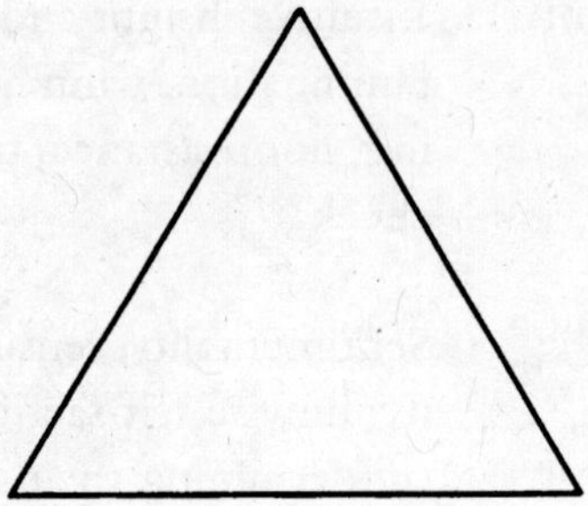

Third Ray

The division of aspects and forces is unreal, except for the purpose of intelligent understanding. . . . This is the will of conditioned purpose.
—Alice A. Bailey

Qualities:	Comprehension, understanding, penetrative and interpretive mental power, adaptability, tact, dignity, impartiality
Type:	Philosopher, scholar, judge, ambassador, diplomat, astrologer
Greatest good/evil:	Understanding/Mental balance
Driving impulse:	To create, understand
Highest attainment:	Comprehension of truth; genius as a result of the overflow of contemplation
Teaching method:	Explanation of principles, impersonal communication, adapting methodology to individual needs

Means of achievement:	Prolonged sequential thinking; right understanding brings right activity; expedience
Weaknesses, vices, or glamours:	Seeing too many sides of an issue; indecision; cruelty, cunning, coldness; intrigue, aloofness, failure to support in a crisis; dilettantism; deliberate and unscrupulous in deceit
Sources of suffering:	Indignity, proven incompetence, darkness
Related religion:	Chaldean, Egyptian
Art:	Literature, poetry, oratory
Gem:	Emerald
Colors:	Green, yellow
Musical note:	"Fa"

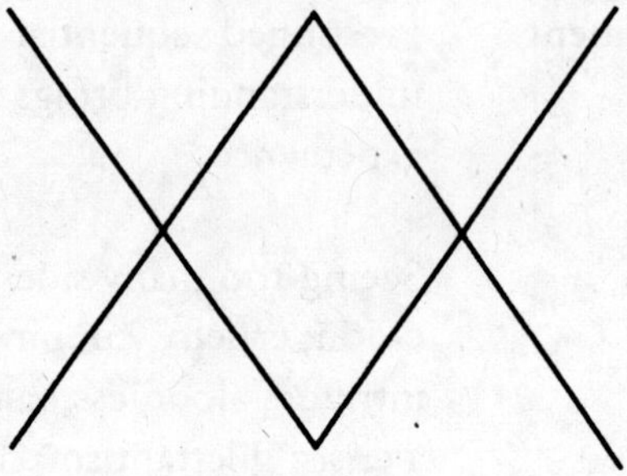

Fourth Ray

This one is the Ray of Harmony . . . it is also Harmony through Conflict. It is a most important ray, for it gives us the clue to the whole problem of pain and suffering.
—Alice A. Bailey

Qualities:	Stability, harmony, balance, beauty, rhythm
Type:	Artist (the medium of expression is influenced by the subray), mediator, interpreter
Greatest good/evil:	Beauty/Ugliness
Driving impulse:	To beautify
Highest attainment:	Harmony, balance, perfect portrayal; perception of the beautiful
Teaching method:	Dramatize; illustrate; elevate through beauty and rhythmic language

Means of achievement:	Dramatization; appeal of beauty and physical perfection; charm
Weaknesses, vices, or glamours:	Alternation, moods of despair and exaltation, sensuousness, posing, self-conceit, self-indulgence
Sources of suffering:	Frustration, failure to express perfectly
Related religion:	Orphic, Egyptian
Art:	Opera
Gem:	Jasper
Colors:	Yellow, bronze-orange
Musical note:	"Mi"

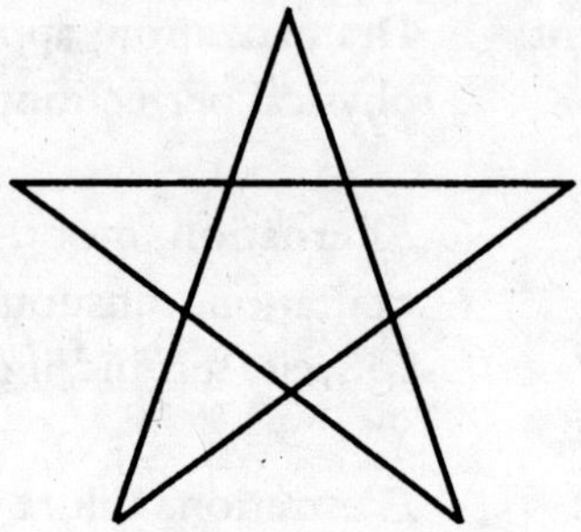

Fifth Ray

This ray . . . is shown to be the revealer of the way . . . a man learns to use all acquired knowledge of the "form divine" in such a way that the inner life is served and the outer becomes the magnetic expression of the divine life.
—Alice A. Bailey

Qualities:	Analytical and logical mentality, accuracy, patience
Type:	Scientist, lawyer, mathematician, alchemist
Greatest good/evil:	Truth, knowledge, fact/Untruth, ignorance, misstatement
Driving impulse:	To discover; thirst for knowledge
Highest attainment:	Knowledge, exhilaration at mental mastery
Teaching method:	Charts, elucidation, diagrams, details; development of accuracy

Means of achievement:	Thinking, seeking, searching, probing, experimenting; patient observation; calculation of facts and accurate deduction
Weaknesses, vices, or glamours:	Smallness of vision, self-centeredness; perceived lack of time; pride, miserliness, criticism, cunning, coldness, one-track mind; pedantic manner, quibbling, curiosity, meanness, separativeness, demanding; accentuating form to the neglect of life
Sources of suffering:	Scorn, mental defeat, fully proven wrong
Related religion:	Zoroastrian
Art:	Painting
Gem:	Topaz
Colors:	Yellow, orange, green
Musical note:	"Re"

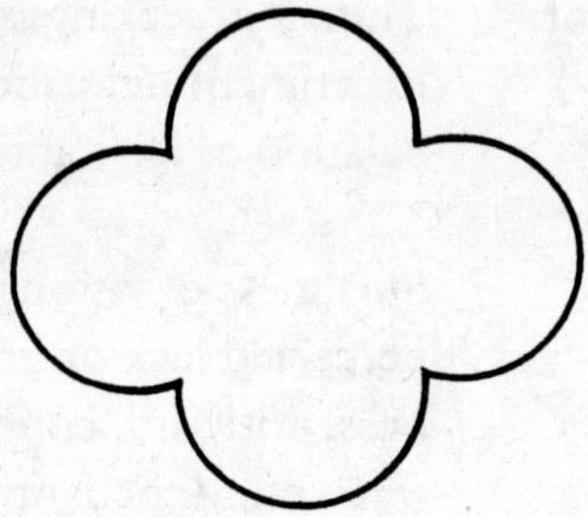

Sixth Ray

It expresses God's desire and is the basic energy emanating from the cosmic astral plane. It conceals the mystery which is to be found in the relationship of the will and desire.
—Alice A. Bailey

Qualities:	One-pointedness, ardor, fiery enthusiasm, devotion, loyalty, sacrificial love
Type:	Saint, mystic, devotee, martyr, evangelist, server, loyal friend
Greatest good/evil:	Unity and a cause, loyalty, fidelity/ Disloyalty, separativeness, individualism
Driving impulse:	To serve and adore; to worship the cause
Highest attainment:	Self-sacrifice; thrill of adoration; martyrdom, service, friendship
Teaching method:	Enkindle, inspire, evoke hero worship

Means of achievement:	One-pointedness
Weaknesses, vices, or glamours:	Overly emotional; impulsiveness, narrowness, intolerance, fanaticism, blind devotion to personalities; tendency to ignore or despise the intellect; sensuality
Sources of suffering:	Disloyalty of those loved and trusted; to be misunderstood and misjudged; melancholy; bruised ideals
Related religion:	Christian
Art:	Architecture (frozen music)
Gem:	Ruby
Colors:	Violet, rose, roseate fire
Musical note:	"Ti"

Seventh Ray

Seventh ray energy is the energy needed to bring order out of chaos and rhythm to replace disorder. It is this energy which will bring in the new world order for which all men wait.
—Alice A. Bailey

Qualities: Grace, precision, ordered beauty, chivalry, dignity, nobility of bearing; orderly method, attention to detail; splendor

Type: Priest, magician, knight, politician, producer, ceremonialist, ritualist

Greatest good/evil: Order/Disorder

Driving impulse: To harness, make manifest

Highest attainment: Ordered splendor, exhilaration at perfect focus from the brow chakra to the physical

Teaching method: Drama; sacred language

Means of achievement:	Ordered synthesis
Weaknesses, vices, or glamours:	Formality, love of office and power; playing politics, using people as tools; bureaucracy, extravagance, regimentation; meticulous and mechanical ceremonialism
Sources of suffering:	Humiliation, loss of outer power and show; frustration, rudeness, discourtesy, adverse criticism by one of lesser importance
Related religion:	Freemasonry, ritualistic aspects of all religions
Art:	Sculpture
Gem:	Amethyst
Colors:	Purple, violet, indigo
Musical note:	"La"

Where are we headed as a culture, a species, a planet? Only time will tell. As of now, it seems clear that in the United States the lens on healing is rapidly changing. Receptivity to new approaches is growing. The often difficult struggle to maintain balance and harmony is persisting despite special-interest pressures to the contrary and a rapidly deteriorating environment.

This tempo of change is apt to gather momentum the closer we move toward a world culture. If we end up forcing those dire outcomes of earth and infrastructure changes predicted so long ago, radionics and radiesthesia will give us powerful tools for self-care. If instead we whirl full speed toward harmony, we may manifest a world in which everyone takes responsibility for their own health and has the freedom to choose whatever supportive method and practitioner they wish. In either instance, your task is simple: delve deeply and creatively into the study of energy patterns, develop your skills in these methods, and *practice*.

Appendix

Techniques for Clearing and Cleansing

Clearing and Resting the Mind

Sri Sathya Sai Baba says there are many dangers inherent in meditation, because most present-day teachers or guides are neither fully realized themselves nor aware of all the pitfalls of this practice. He adds that today the only genuine guide is God and the one safe technique is the Jyoti meditation—an ancient method of focusing on divine light by way of a candle flame.

The Jyoti Meditation

- Pray to God, or whoever you perceive as supreme and absolute, to accept and guide your meditation.
- Sitting comfortably, with a straight spine, look at the flame of a candle through partially closed eyes.
- Keep gazing at the flame until your breathing becomes slow and regular.
- Continue gazing at the flame until you are able to visualize it with your eyes shut.
- Through visualization, bring the light down from your brow into your heart; imagine the heart's lotus petals opening, purifying all your thoughts and emotions. Then move the light throughout your body, allowing its illumination to dispel all darkness within

you. Each time you move the light of this pure flame, a cleansing is taking place in that area.

- Now move the flame to bless friends, family, and the world.
- Bringing the flame back, center it in your heart and continue to sit quietly.
- Send love and gratitude to God.

> *Meditation is the name for the period of rest we provide for the busy and wayward mind.*
>
> —Sri Sathya Sai Baba

Cleansing the Physical Body and Foods

We seem assaulted on every side today by substances that are harmful to the human body. Even organic gardens fail to protect our produce from the effects of debilitating pollutants. The so-called safe tap water we drink often contains toxic residues from spills, dumping, or seepage. More and more examples of residential toxic-waste contamination are surfacing. In addition to raising a public outcry against the condition of our environment, we can approach a state of more balanced well-being by taking precautions with our bodies and the foods we eat.

Baths or soaks can effectively clean out the toxic residues from metallics, radiation, and pesticides. One highly therapeutic ingredient to add to the bathwater is plain old-fashioned *Clorox*. For decades Peace Corps personnel living in remote areas have used this product to purify water. According to biochemists, Clorox oxidizes free sulfhydryl groups—potential radical formers—into disulfides, thereby impeding their destructive action. Clorox can safely be used to clean the body and to remove some of the hazardous pollutants that may accumulate on produce during its journey from seed to the consumer. A 3 percent grade of *hydrogen peroxide* (H_2O_2) will serve the same purposes. Homeopathic preparations, too, can help rid the body of toxic metals. The following four cleansing methods are both easy and effective.

Body Soak for Removal of Metallics

Many people take this bath as a matter of course to counteract their everyday exposures to aluminum, mercury, or other toxic metals. It is best taken before going to bed at night.

- Add 1 cup of plain Clorox (in Europe use Javelle Wasser 7%) to a full tub of water as hot as can be withstood.
- Soak for at least 30 minutes or until the water cools to body temperature.
- Air dry.
- In the morning, rinse.

Body Soak for Removal of Radiation

This bath helps neutralize hyperacidity resulting from exposure to X rays or other forms of radiation. As with the Clorox soak, it is best taken before going to bed at night.

- Add 1 pound of sea salt and 1 pound of baking soda (bicarbonate of soda) to a full tub of water as hot as can be withstood.
- Soak for at least 30 minutes or until the water cools to body temperature.
- Air dry.
- In the morning, rinse.

In times of exposure to *significant* levels of radiation, also try this drink.

- Add 1 teaspoon of sea salt and 1 teaspoon of baking soda to 1 quart of *distilled* water.
- Mix well and divide into four 8-ounce glasses.
- Drink the first glass of fluid, then an hour later drink the second glass.
- Wait two hours before drinking the third glass of fluid, then another two hours before drinking the fourth glass.
- If more of this solution is needed to neutralize symptoms, space the additional drinks three hours apart.

(*Note:* For additional protection, take 3 calcium lactate tablets with each drink.)

Body Soak for Removal of Pollutants

Baths prepared with Epsom salts, herbs, or apple cider vinegar help draw out pollutants. Apple cider vinegar soaks are highly recommended after exposures to carbon monoxide.

(*Note:* In natural healing programs that assist the body in ridding itself of toxins and poisons accumulated over time, reactions are common. Most often, these take the form of rashes and other skin eruptions, chills, or fever. Occasionally, discolored bathwater has been reported following instances of extreme toxicity.)

Cleansing Bath for Fruits and Vegetables

This treatment not only detoxifies produce but enhances its appearance and staying power as well. The treatment was used as the basis for an extensive cleansing and detoxification program developed at Sierra States University School of Nutrition in California, after which it was adopted by other organizations that reported excellent results.

- Add one-half (½) teaspoon of plain Clorox to 1 gallon of water.
- Soak thin-skinned or leafy fruits and vegetables in this solution for 10 minutes. For thick-skinned or root produce, soak for 15–20 minutes.
- Remove the fruits and vegetables; rinse in clean water for 10–15 minutes; then dry and store.

(*Note:* Vegetables that are left soaking for too long are apt to become limp and discolored from oxidation, so be sure to adhere to the stated soak and rinse times. And do not use more Clorox than directed.)

Glossary

Allopathic. Based on the traditional Western medical model of treating disease with medicines that are different from the condition itself.

Attar. A pure essential oil used to activate the body's healing processes.

Chakra. Sanskrit for "wheel"; a subtle energy channel along the spine.

Chromotherapy. A healing modality based on color.

Critical rotation position (CRP). The correct orientation for a witness; used in "tuning" a broadcast.

Electromagnetic frequency (EMF). The number of oscillations per second of an electromagnetic wave that in the body's energy field is subject to influence by outside forces.

Etheric body (also known as vital body). A subtle vehicle that encloses and interpenetrates the physical body, emitting energy that holds together the personality.

Homeopathy. An energy medicine that heals by strengthening the body's own vital-force mechanism via dilute remedies which in larger doses produce symptoms similar to those they are mitigating.

Kirlian photography. A photographic technique that captures the energy fields radiating from living things.

Life-field (L-field). An energy field that seems to precede the existence of the physical form to which it corresponds.

Miasm. A predisposition toward chronic disease resulting from the etheric body's absorption of tainted energy from the earth's etheric field.

Nadis. Sanskrit for "motion"; subtle channels forming an etheric nervous network of conduits for the flow of life-force energy.

Organizational field (O-field). An energy field that surrounds the universe and emanates from the Creator, or higher mind.

Polarity. The harmonious interplay of positively and negatively charged forces.

Prana. Sanskrit for "life force."

Pranamonics. A new system of healing that simultaneously treats body, mind, and spirit.

Radiations. The energy waves emanating from all things.

Radiesthesia (also known as dowsing). Use of a pendulum for ascertaining analyses of and remedies for ailments.

Radionics. A method of healing at a distance by way of instrumentation and enhanced perceptions.

Rae cards. A series of treatment cards based on geometric patterns.

Rates. Units of measurement indicated on the dials of radionic instruments and set before and throughout a treatment.

Sanjeevini. A prayer-based Vedantic healing system that employs spiritual diagrams to infuse divine healing powers into substances.

Seven cosmic rays. The building forces of all things in the manifested universe.

Thought field (T-field). An energy field that is believed to influence healing by attaching itself to matter.

Witness. A sample—lock of hair, blood spot, sputum, urine specimen, photograph, or original signature—that carries the vibration of the subject receiving analysis or treatment.

Resources

BOOKS AND PERIODICALS

Radionics

Baerlain, E., and L. Dower. *Healing with Radionics.* Wellingborough, England: Thorsons Publishers, 1980. Available from The Keys College of Radionics, PO Box 194, London SE16 1Q2, England.

Mason, Keith. *Radionics and Progressive Energies.* Essex, England: C. W. Daniel Company, 1984.

Paris, Don. *Regaining Wholeness through the Subtle Dimensions.* Stanwood, WA: Living from Vision, 1993.

Radionic Journal. Available from The Secretary, The Radionic Association and The School of Radionics, Baerlein House, Goose Green, Deddington, Banbury, Oxon 0X15 0SZ, England.

Russell, Edward W. *Report on Radionics.* Suffolk, England: Neville Spearman, 1973.

Tansley, David V. *Chakras, Rays and Radionics.* Essex, England: C. W. Daniel Company, 1984; *Dimensions of Radionics.* N. Devon, England: Health Science Press, 1977; *Radionics and the Subtle Anatomy of Man.* N. Devon England: Health Science Press, 1972; and *The Raiment of Light.* London, England: Routledge and Kegan Paul, 1984.

Radiesthesia

Blackburn, Gabriele. *The Science and Art of the Pendulum.* Ojai, CA: Idylwild Books, 1983.

Graves, Tom. *The Elements of Pendulum Dowsing,* Dorset, England: Element Books, 1989.

Mermet, Abbé. *Principles and Practice of Radiesthesia.* London, England: Robinson & Watkins Books, 1959.

Richards, W. Guyon. *The Chain of Life.* Essex, England: C. W. Daniel Company, 1'954.

Tomlinson, H. *The Use of the Pendulum in Medicine.* London, England: Medical Society for the Study of Radiesthesia.

Wethered, V. D. *An Introduction to Medical Radiesthesia and Radionics.* Devon, England: Health Science Press.

Esoteric Philosophy

Bailey, Alice A. *Esoteric Healing, Esoteric Psychology,* vols. 1 & 2, *A Treatise on Cosmic Fire,* and *A Treatise on White Magic.* New York: Lucis Publishing Company, 1979, 1982.

Eastcott, Michal J. *The Story of Self.* Wheaton, IL: Theosophical Publishing House, 1980.

Gerber, Richard. *Vibrational Medicine: New Choices for Healing Ourselves.* Santa Fe, NM: Bear & Co., 1988.

Hall, Manly P. *Man: Grand Symbol of the Mysteries.* Los Angeles: Philosophical Research Society, 1972.

Hunt, Valerie V. *Infinite Mind: The Science of Human Vibrations.* Malibu, CA: Malibu Publication Company, 1989.

Joy, W. Brugh, *Joy's Way.* Boston: Houghton Mifflin Company, 1979.

Jurriaanse, Aart. *Bridges.* Cape, South Africa: Sun Centre School of Esoteric Philosophy, 1978.

Parrish-Harra, Carol E. *Adventure in Meditation: Spirituality for the 21st Century,* vols. 1, 2, 3. Tahlequah, OK: Sparrow Hawk Press, 1997.

Study Group. *Spirituality and Science.* Bombay, India: Sri Sathya Sai Baba Trust, 1985.

Zambucka, Kristin. *Ano Ano, the Seed.* Honolulu, HI: Mano Publishing, 1978.

Patterns

Westlake, Aubrey T. *The Pattern of Health.* London, England: Shamballa, 1973.

Aromatherapy

Tisserand, Robert B. *The Art of Aromatherapy.* New York: Destiny Books, 1977.

Young, Gary D. *An Introduction to Young Living Essential Oils and Aromatherapy.* Salt Lake City, UT: Essential Press Publishing, 1996.

Color Therapy

Bhattacharya, B. *VIBGYOR: The Science of Cosmic Ray Therapy.* India: Good Companions, 1957.

Brennan, Barbara Ann. *Light Emerging: The Journey of Personal Healing.* New York: Bantam Books, 1993.

Clark, Linda. *The Ancient Art of Color Healing.* New York: Pocketbooks, 1976.

Copen, Bruce. *A Rainbow of Health.* W. Sussex, England: Academic Publications, 1975.

Heline, Corinne. *Color and Music in the New Age.* Marina del Rey, CA: DeVorss & Company, 1964.

Hunt, Roland. *Seven Keys to Color Healing.* London, England: C. W. Daniel Company, 1971.

Ott, John N. *Health and Light.* New York: Pocketbooks, 1976.

Gem Remedies

Cayce, Edgar. *Gems and Stones.* Virginia Beach, VA: A.R.E. Press, 1976.

Gurudas. *Gem Elixirs and Vibrational Healing,* vol. 2. Boulder, CO: Cassandra Press, 1985.

Mella, Dorothee L., with Michelle Lusson. *Gem Pharmacy.* Albuquerque, NM: Domel Tote-a-Book, 1992.

Homeopathy and Cell Salts

Bhattacharya, A. K. *Eclectic Medicine.* Calcutta, India: Firma KLM Private, Ltd., 1984.

Boericke, William. *Homeopathic Materia Medica.* Philadelphia: Boericke & Runyon, 1927.

Boericke, William, and W. A. Dewey. *The Twelve Tissue Remedies of Schüssler,* 6th ed. New Delhi, India: B. Jain Publishing Private Ltd., 1985.

Cummings, Stephen, and Dana Ullman. *Everybody's Guide to Homeopathic Medicines.* Boston: Houghton Mifflin Company, 1984.

Shepherd, Dorothy. *Homeopathy for the First Aider.* Essex, England: Health Science Press, 1980.

Vithoulkas, George. *The Science of Homeopathy.* New York: Grove Press, 1980.

The Seven Rays

Baker, Douglas. *The Seven Rays: Keys to the Mysteries.* Wellingborough, England: Thorsons Publishing Group, 1977.

Eastcott, Michal J. *The Seven Rays of Energy.* Tunbridge Wells, England: Sundial House, 1980.

Hodson, Geoffrey. *The 7 Human Temperaments.* Adyar, Madras, India: Theosophical Publishing House, 1977.

Index

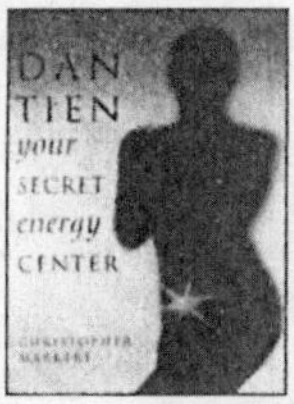

DAN TIEN: Your Secret Energy Center— *Christopher Markert*

The Dan-Tien is a source of primal wisdom and vital energy that resides within each of us. For thousands of years people in the East have learned to gather life energy (*ch'i*) in this center to promote well-being and longevity. *Dan Tien: Your Secret Energy Center* reveals the secrets of the Dan-Tien to you in a friendly manner.

ISBN: 81-7822-212-4

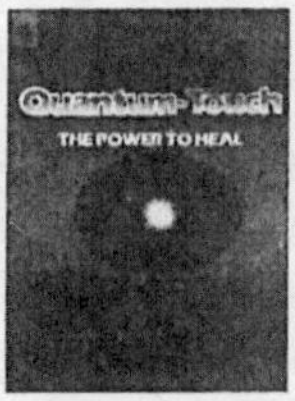

QUANTUM-TOUCH: The Power to Heal — *Richard Gordon*

The book represents a major breakthrough in the art of hands-on healing and teaches you to use special breathing and body focusing techniques to raise your energy level so high that with a light touch you can see postural corrections spontaneously occur as bones gently glide back into their correct alignment. Beyond this, pain and inflammation are rapidly reduced.

ISBN: 81-7822-009-1

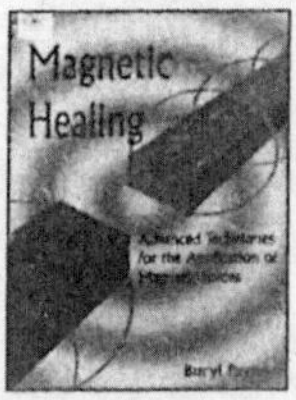

MAGNETIC HEALING — *Buryl Payne*

Discover the positive benefits of magnetism for improving your health and well-being. The book narrates: What ailments can be treated with magnets • How do magnets work to heal the body • Which polarity should be used for which condition • What is the correct way to use magnets • How long should magnets be placed on the body • What are the latest magnetic health products now being used; etc.

ISBN: 81-7822-002-4

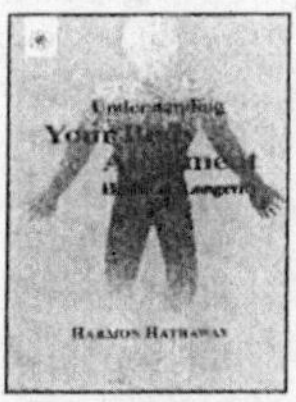

UNDERSTANDING YOUR BODY ALIGNMENT: Health and Longevity — *Harmon Hathaway*

The book offers very effective techniques for releasing tension and frozen energy, helping the body to function fully. It helps to reach the sacred point of confluence of mind, body and spirit in holistic perspective. It can provide a direct natural solution to many human illnesses, especially those related to: Emphysema, Asthma, Lung diseases, Bursitis, Tendonitis and Arthritis, etc.

ISBN: 81-7822-001-6

BOOKS OF RELATED INTEREST

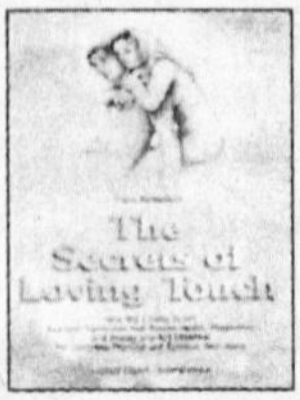

THE SECRETS OF LOVING TOUCH : How the Loving Touch Releases Beneficial and Essential Hormones — *Franz Benedikter*

By gently touching certain body zones, relaxing, activating and euphoretic hormones are released which benefit health, happiness, and beauty and are essential for complete physical and spiritual well-being. This very effective program introduces a new age of tenderness.

ISBN: 81-7822-211-6

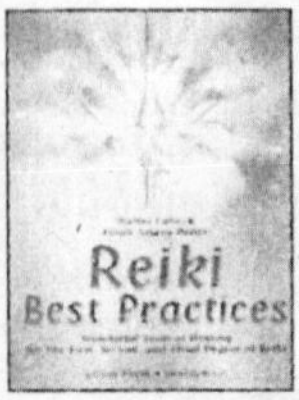

REIKI—BEST PRACTICES: Wonderful Tools of Healing—*Walter Lübeck & Frank Arjava Petter*

Reiki is always flowing, naturally and continuously even without us doing anything at all help it. With good instructions and special techniques to support the process it can flow in a more focused way. These methods are extremely helpful in working effectively with Reiki.

ISBN: 81-7822-209-4

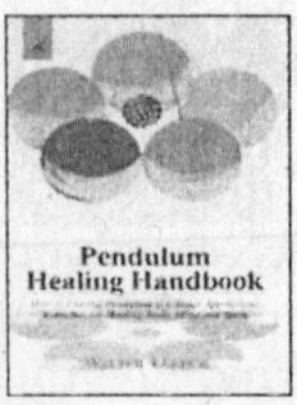

PENDULUM HEALING HANDBOOK: How to Use Pendulum to Choose Appropriate Remedies for Healing Body, Mind and Spirit—*W. Lśbeck*

It answers the questions that normally occur following a person's first experiences with the pendulum. It explains the selection of the right pendulum, shows the correct way to hold it, and also explains the possibilities of energetic cleansing.

ISBN: 81-7822-003-2

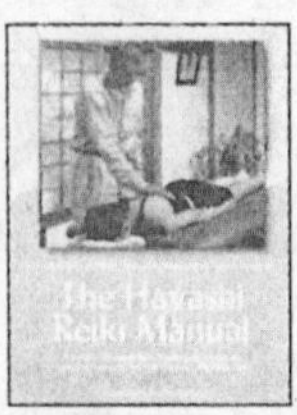

THE HAYASHI REIKI MANUAL: Traditional Japanese Healing Techniques from the Founder of the Western Reiki System — *F.A. Petter, Tadao Yamaguchi* and *Chujiro Hayashi*

This manual consists of: • The story of Dr. Chujiro Hayashi • Main exercises of the Hayashi Reiki system • The blood circulation technique • Specific documents such as the original certificates of Dr. Hayashi • Colorful sequence of photos.

ISBN: 81-7822-210-8